DR. THOMSON'S 1895 CORRESPONDENCE COURSE

IN OPTICS.

DR. THOMSON'S
1895 CORRESPONDENCE COURSE
IN
OPTICS.

WITH HISTORICAL COMMENTARY

BY

MONROE J. HIRSCH, O.D., Ph.D.

SCHOOL OF OPTOMETRY, UNIVERSITY OF CALIFORNIA

BERKELEY, CALIFORNIA

PROFESSIONAL PRESS, INC.

CHICAGO, ILLINOIS

© 1975 by Professional Press, Inc.

FIRST PRINTING

ISBN-0-87873-017-6

Library of Congress Catalog Card Number: 74-31552

Published by Professional Press, Inc.
Chicago, Illinois 60611

Printed in the U.S.A.

INTRODUCTION.

I N February and March 1899 an advertisement for the South Bend College of Optics appeared in *The Optical Journal Supplement,* a monthly magazine for opticians. The advertisement, signed by Dr. H. A. Thomson, president of the college, describes a correspondence course in "the optical science." The tuition fee for the course, described as "a complete course of instruction," was $25.00. Although the subject matter is termed "optics," the material that was covered would be known today as optometry.[1] A student, if he wished, could take the same course in residence at the college for a $50.00 tuition fee. This advertisement and two others that appeared in the same year in *The Optical Journal Supplement* are reproduced in Figs. 1, 2 and 3.

In 1973, the bulletins issued by any of the 12 colleges of optometry in the United States or the two in Canada describe the course of instruction in optometry as requiring four years of professional school after two years of basic science courses[2] at the undergraduate college level. During the 1972–73 academic year, the mean tuition fee at the six independent colleges of optometry in the United States[3] was $1952 (range, $1826 to $2135); at the six state-supported universities, the mean tuition fee was $851 for residents (range, $136 to $1600) and $1850 for non-residents of the state (range, $1360 to $2108). Thus, tuition for all those except residents attending their own state university was approximately $2000.

In the three quarters of a century during which the optometric profession developed in the United States, the time required for formal education increased almost one hundred fold from a few weeks to between six and eight years; the cost of educating an optometrist increased approximately eighty fold. With such tremendous increases in cost and time required, how much change occurred in the content of the curriculum in optometry? The correspondence course of Dr. Thomson offers an excellent description of the content of optometry at the beginning of its modern history in the United States—especially since the same material was the basis for the in-residence course at the South Bend College of Optics.

The complete text of the Thomson course on optics is reproduced in this volume. It was copyrighted in 1895, and was widely used for approximately 15 years thereafter. Since the Thomson course contains all that a student was required to learn when optometry began, comparing it to today's body of knowledge serves as a measure of the increase in optometric content during the first three quarters of a century of its history. The student of optometry today uses a minimum of 25 textbooks during his college training. One book alone, the definitive textbook on Clinical Refraction by Irvin M. Borish published in 1970[4] contains

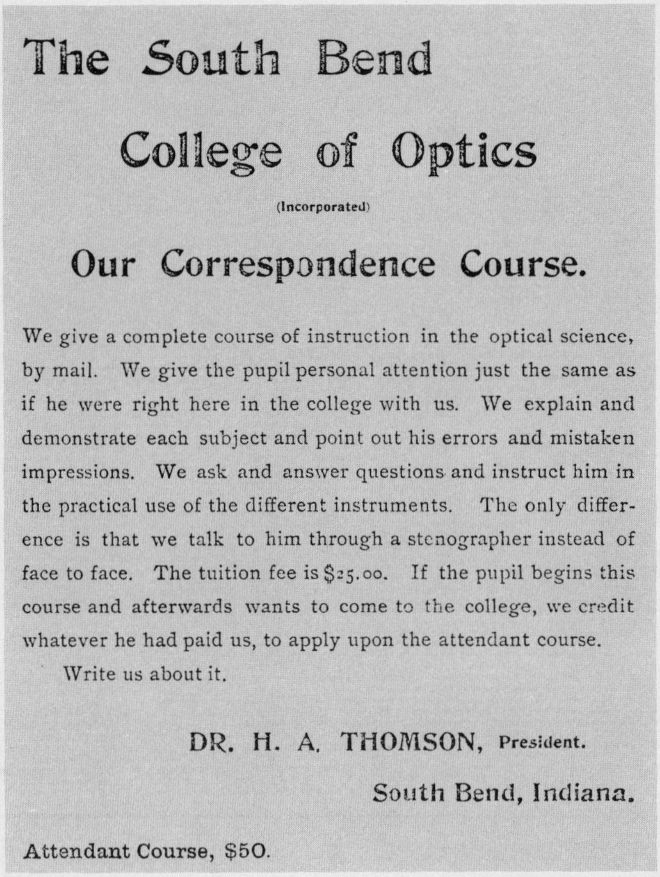

The South Bend

College of Optics

(Incorporated)

Our Correspondence Course.

We give a complete course of instruction in the optical science, by mail.   We give the pupil personal attention just the same as if he were right here in the college with us.   We explain and demonstrate each subject and point out his errors and mistaken impressions.   We ask and answer questions and instruct him in the practical use of the different instruments.   The only difference is that we talk to him through a stenographer instead of face to face.   The tuition fee is $25.00.   If the pupil begins this course and afterwards wants to come to the college, we credit whatever he had paid us, to apply upon the attendant course.

   Write us about it.

DR. H. A. THOMSON, President.

South Bend, Indiana.

Attendant Course, $50.

FIG. 1

more than ten times the amount of material in the Thomson course. During his four years of professional school training, the student today writes more words in his many mid-term and final examination papers than the total number of words in the Thomson course!

   The Thomson course reproduced in this volume was by no means the only course in optometry at the turn of the century. Just prior to the licensing of optometrists early in the 20th century many opticians learned to test vision either by apprenticeship, by one or two week residence courses (usually given by a single teacher), by self study, by home correspondence courses, or by a combination of these.

Many opticians decided to enter the field of vision testing in the United States in the last decade of the nineteenth century. The first university-affiliated optometric college, that at Columbia University in New York, was not established until 1910. Thus, between 1890 and 1910 many opticians wished to learn vision testing and there was no shortage of persons willing to teach them. During this period, no fewer than 60 proprietary courses or schools of optics flourished. The length of the course was anywhere from a few days to a few weeks. Usually the faculty consisted of one individual (whose name was given to the course or school) who himself practiced vision testing and conducted classes on a part time basis in his office. The students were oculists (eye physicians) or opticians who wished to learn vision testing. Often both oculists and opticians attended the same schools and learned to test vision in the same classes.

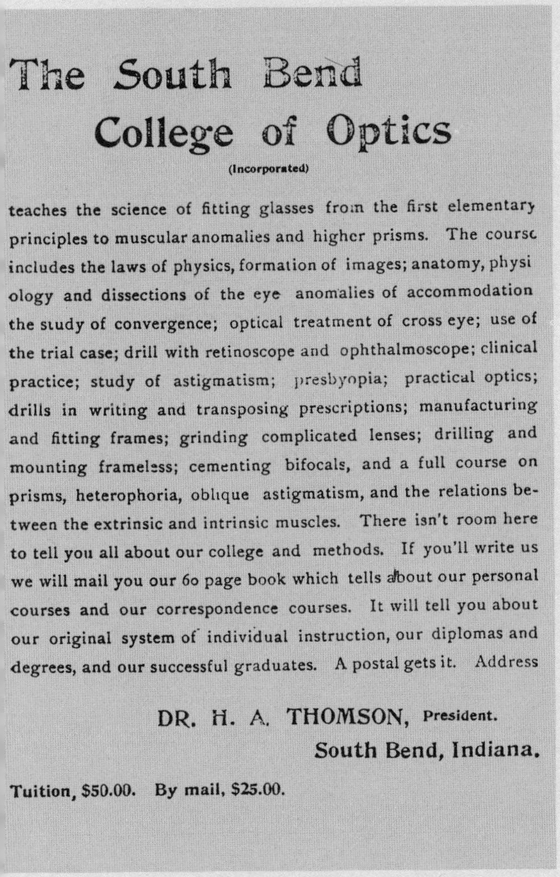

The South Bend College of Optics

(Incorporated)

teaches the science of fitting glasses from the first elementary principles to muscular anomalies and higher prisms. The course includes the laws of physics, formation of images; anatomy, physiology and dissections of the eye anomalies of accommodation the study of convergence; optical treatment of cross eye; use of the trial case; drill with retinoscope and ophthalmoscope; clinical practice; study of astigmatism; presbyopia; practical optics; drills in writing and transposing prescriptions; manufacturing and fitting frames; grinding complicated lenses; drilling and mounting frameless; cementing bifocals, and a full course on prisms, heterophoria, oblique astigmatism, and the relations between the extrinsic and intrinsic muscles. There isn't room here to tell you all about our college and methods. If you'll write us we will mail you our 60 page book which tells about our personal courses and our correspondence courses. It will tell you about our original system of individual instruction, our diplomas and degrees, and our successful graduates. A postal gets it. Address

DR. H. A. THOMSON, President.

South Bend, Indiana.

Tuition, $50.00. By mail, $25.00.

FIG. 2

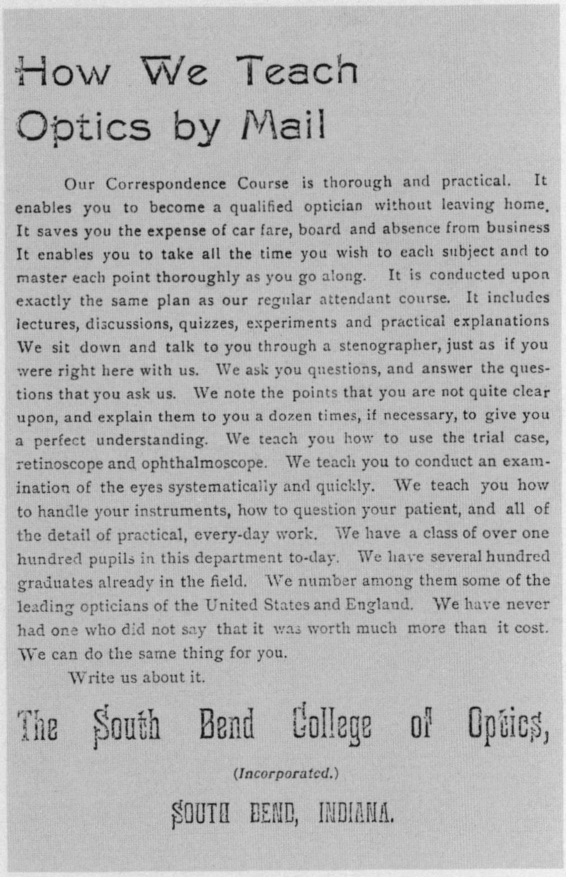

How We Teach Optics by Mail

Our Correspondence Course is thorough and practical. It enables you to become a qualified optician without leaving home. It saves you the expense of car fare, board and absence from business It enables you to take all the time you wish to each subject and to master each point thoroughly as you go along. It is conducted upon exactly the same plan as our regular attendant course. It includes lectures, discussions, quizzes, experiments and practical explanations We sit down and talk to you through a stenographer, just as if you were right here with us. We ask you questions, and answer the questions that you ask us. We note the points that you are not quite clear upon, and explain them to you a dozen times, if necessary, to give you a perfect understanding. We teach you how to use the trial case, retinoscope and ophthalmoscope. We teach you to conduct an examination of the eyes systematically and quickly. We teach you how to handle your instruments, how to question your patient, and all of the detail of practical, every-day work. We have a class of over one hundred pupils in this department to-day. We have several hundred graduates already in the field. We number among them some of the leading opticians of the United States and England. We have never had one who did not say that it was worth much more than it cost. We can do the same thing for you.

Write us about it.

The South Bend College of Optics,

(Incorporated.)

SOUTH BEND, INDIANA.

FIG. 3

Two present day schools of optometry evolved from early one man courses intended initially for physicians and later for both physicians and opticians. The Southern California College of Optometry was initially the Los Angeles School of Ophthalmology and Optometry run by M. B. Ketchum who practiced eye, ear, nose, and throat medicine when he was not teaching vision testing at his school. The Illinois College of Optometry had its start as the Northern Illinois College of Ophthalmology and Otology, organized in 1872 by Drs. George W. and J. B. McFatrich; physicians were taught sight testing on Sunday mornings for many years and in 1898 opticians were admitted to the classes.

Between 1890 and 1910 one or two week courses in vision testing were offered by several manufacturers of optical equipment. The course was part of a program of selling trial lens sets and other vision testing equipment. The Spencer Optical Manufacturing Company offered a two week course for $25 tuition and introduced the students to the Audemaire Trial Case of Test Lenses. The Julius King Optical Company offered a brief course in vision testing at its offices in New York City and Cleveland. This course lasted one week and introduced the student to the Elite Test Case and Optician's Outfit, supplied by King with the course.

Modern optometry, at present the third largest primary health care providing profession in the United States, evolved from such meager beginnings. A subject taught by individual physicians on Sunday mornings, or in one week correspondence courses, or in two-week in-residence "colleges," or by manufacturers of optical equipment as part of their sales program for optical testing equipment grew to a body of knowledge whose mastery now requires six or more years of college training; and this change occurred within the customary three score and ten years of an individual lifetime.

The Thomson Correspondence Course is typical of the courses given at the early colleges, by manufacturers, and by individuals in the period just before regular colleges of optometry were established. To appreciate the Thomson manuscript fully, the reader should have certain historical information, and this will be supplied in this introduction.

Vision Testing Prior to the 1900's.

When spectacles were invented in Europe toward the end of the 13th century, a new occupation emerged—that of fabricating and supplying spectacles. For about 500 years thereafter, spectacle-makers (later called opticians) supplied members of the public with spectacles. During the early years of this half millenium, spectacles were fabricated in small workshops or factories and were sold by peddlers or by the operators of retail shops that sold other merchandise (haberdashers, for example). Later in this period, particularly during the 18th and 19th centuries, the fabrication and the sale of spectacles (and other optical devices such as telescopes and microscopes) were carried out in the same shop. The proprietors of these shops, the opticians, were skilled craftsmen and were the predecessors of today's optometrists.

By the time America was colonized, opticianry was a thriving craft and recognized guild in England and several European countries. Among those who came to America were some opticians and they set up shops on the new continent particularly in the major population centers. By the time the United States attained its independence, several opticians owned shops in American cities. Here, they manufactured and sold spectacles, telescopes, microscopes and other optical devices just as opticians in England and Continental European countries were doing.

The spectacles that the early opticians offered were prefabricated and were not made for a specific patient. The lenses of early spectacles were convex or concave spheres and were of equal power for the right and left eyes. Since there were only a few dozen spherical lens powers customarily used, it was possible to make spectacles in advance and then allow the customer to select from a tray of ready-made spectacles that pair that seemed to help him the most.[5] The optician sometimes helped the customer to select an appropriate pair of spectacles, but the amount of help was minimal. The customer usually made his choice after trying on several pairs of spectacles from a tray or two, each containing a dozen or so pairs of ready-made spectacles.

During the 19th century, knowledge of lenses and of the eye and its anomalies became markedly more sophisticated. Opticians learned to make cylindrical lenses for the correction of astigmatism. They learned that the lens required by an individual's right eye was not always the same as that required by the left eye. They also learned how to make spectacles that had two different focal powers, making it possible for an individual to have a lens for distance viewing and another lens for near viewing incorporated in a single pair of spectacles. Opticians also learned that a spectacle lens not only focussed light but that it could displace an image through prismatic power—and they noted that some patients benefited by the inclusion of prismatic components in their spectacles.

The result of these discoveries in the characteristics of spectacles, i.e., that the lenses could be different for each eye, that lenses could be made with two foci, with cylinders, and with prismatic power, was to increase the number of possible pairs of spectacles from a few dozen to an almost infinite number. The prefabrication of spectacles was no longer desirable. Spectacles had to be made to order for each patient—and if lenses were to be made for the needs of one individual alone, tests had to be performed to determine the specific lens to be placed before each of his eyes.

During the last half of the nineteenth century, too, methods of testing vision to determine an optimal spectacle lens were developed. Knowledge about the eye and its anomalies was advanced markedly during this period. The classical work of Helmholtz on physiological optics and of Donders on the clinical application of physiological optics in correcting vision anomalies were both published in the 1860's. During the last half of the nineteenth century, the retinoscope, the ophthalmoscope, test types, and the keratometer were invented—all tools needed to test a patient's vision.

Thus, toward the end of the nineteenth century the groundwork had been laid for a new way of supplying spectacles. Technical discoveries and improvements in opticianry made it possible to fabricate spectacles specifically for individual patients. Basic knowledge about the visual system and its needs for correction of its anomalies had been supplied by such giants as Hemholtz and Donders. Instruments for testing vision and eyes to determine the specific lens needed by an individual were at hand. But who would do the testing of vision? The time was ready for a new occupation to emerge or for an existing occupation to increase its scope to include vision testing. If an existing occupation were to take on the task of examining eyes for spectacles, it would be either the opticians who, for 500 years, had been fabricating spectacles or the oculists, eye physicians who were already knowledgeable about the eye and were treating its disease through medication and surgery.

By the last decade of the 19th century, a few of the best opticians and some oculists were already testing vision. But, neither opticians nor oculists were ideally trained to take on the task. Moreover there was no clear agreement among opticians nor among oculists as to what their role should be in the field of vision care. Yet, technology was at a point where vision testing for individually designed spectacles was ready. Knowledge of physiological optics, instrumentation for sight-testing, techniques for fabricating spectacles were all at a point where the job could be done. But who would do the job?

Both opticians and oculists lacked some of the training needed to become the vision testing profession. Oculists, trained as physicians, understood the biological sciences, medicine and surgery, but were usually less well trained in optics, mathematics and physical sciences. Moreover, the eye physician's major interest was usually in the biological aspects of the eye rather than in the physical aspects of lenses and optics. Most important, there was a long tradition among eye physicians of discouraging the use of spectacles. Until the time of Donders (1864) most eye physicians had warned patients of the supposedly harmful effects of wearing spectacles. Even oculists who did not oppose the use of spectacles did not prescribe them. Rather, they sent their patients to an optician to select a pair of spectacles—often with the admonition that these not be worn too frequently. A few physicians did recognize the value of spectacles, did test vision and prescribe lenses, but they were in the minority.

Donders, himself an eye physician, is usually referred to as the "Father of Scientific Refraction." He placed the testing of vision and the specifying of spectacles for individuals on a scientific basis, and some oculists followed his teaching. But the long tradition of the physician against prescribing spectacles had its effect. Even though the young oculist was exposed to the work of Donders, those in practice prior to 1870 would not have been trained to do sight-testing. Late in the 19th and early in the 20th century those physicians who believed that oculists should test vision to determine spectacles for patients became more and more frantic in their warnings to their colleagues. They pointed out that if oculists did not test for spectacles some other group (opticians, for example) would begin to do so.

Interestingly, despite the negative attitude toward the use of spectacles by physicians before Donders, much of the science and art of vision testing was developed by eye physicians. Those physicians who did have aptitude and skill in mathematics and the physical sciences, like Donders and Helmholtz, did develop both techniques and instruments for sight testing. But the old attitudes and the lack of interest on the part of most oculists persisted and militated against oculists becoming the group that could care for the needs of the public in the area of vision care that required optical devices.

Just as there were factors that militated against the eye physicians of the late nineteenth century filling the need of the public for an occupation that would test vision and design spectacles for the neutralization of anomalies of refraction and accommodation, there were also negative factors that affected the opticians. Opticians understood mathematics and optics and had the skills in working with lenses and spectacles. They had a 500 year tradition of spectacle making and of supplying spectacles to the public. Most of the advances in practical ophthalmic optics had been the work of opticians. The design and fabrication of cylindrical lenses for the neutralization of astigmatism, of bifocals, and of the prismatic aspect of lenses had all been developed by opticians and were familiar to most opticians. However, most opticians had little formal schooling, having learned their craft through apprenticeship. If oculists were weak in mathematics and optics, the opticians were equally deficient in biological science. Often self-taught, most opticians had a good knowledge of optics, the action of lenses, and the physical sciences needed to understand optics; they had little or no knowledge of anatomy, physiology, and the biological sciences needed to master physiological optics. If the attitude of physicians had been to deprecate the use of spectacles the attitude of opticians had been to make and sell spectacles but not to test vision. Opticians were essentially craftsmen and merchants; the concept of serving in a consulting position was foreign to most of them. Many opticians resisted increasing their scope to include vision testing, and in fact, many never did adopt this new function, remaining always makers and suppliers of spectacles to the order and specifications of another.

In 1890, neither opticians as a group nor oculists as a group were adequately trained or philosophically oriented toward filling a need that had developed. But there were individuals in each group who were qualified, and who recognized the need. Instruments and techniques for sight testing were developed by individual physicians; sight testing was performed by some physicians who followed the teachings of Donders, and these physicians also added to the fund of knowledge and taught oculists and opticians. Opticians with better than average training developed new lens products, increased their understanding of optics, and also in their own practices engaged in vision testing. Opticians like the McAllisters in Philadelphia, a family group, some member of which had practiced opticianry in America since the 1700's, had been testing vision as early as 1870, and taught other opticians and oculists to test vision. Charles Prentice of New York, trained in Germany in optics, and a contributor to knowledge in optics, had been testing vision prior to 1890 and advocated that other opticians do so. It was, in fact, the accusation that in testing vision *and charging for the service* Prentice was practicing medicine that started him on his crusade to obtain legal recognition for opticians as vision testers.

Clearly, by 1890, the situation in the eye testing field was chaotic. On the one hand, eye physicians, who traditionally had opposed the use of spectacles, were adopting the knowledge developed by Helmholtz and Donders. Eye physicians, not specifically trained nor licensed to test vision, were being urged, by those within the group who recognized the public's need, to adopt the function of sight tester. Opticians, on the other hand, members of a 500 year old craft and knowledgeable in optics, were also not specifically licensed to test vision. They too were being urged by members of their group, who recognized the developing need for sight testing for spectacles, to broaden the scope of their practice.

In the chaos of the late 19th century, a large number of "crash" courses designed to teach sight testing to oculists and/or opticians were developed. It was in this environment that courses like that of Dr. Thomson were developed. Technology had made sight testing for spectacles necessary. Neither of the occupations involved in vision care, opticians and oculists, had the needed training. Courses were developed to teach large numbers of people how to test vision and design spectacles for the individual visual system.

Dr. Thomson's Correspondence Course in Optics.

Dr. H. A. Thomson prepared and copyrighted (1895) the series of lessons that were used in his correspondence course and at the South Bend College of Optics, of which Dr. Thomson was administrator and faculty. Dr. Thomson stated in his advertisements that the correspondence course was the same as the course given at the college, the only difference being that he would be talking to the student "through a stenographer instead of face to face."

The teaching method of having a formal series of lessons through which the student proceeded was widely used in the late 19th and early 20th century. Carel C. Koch has described the course at the DeMars College of Optometry in Minneapolis at the time of World War I, as consisting of a series of lectures given during a single semester. The same lectures were repeated every semester, and the student was required to listen to the same lectures four times. Thus, although the course required two years, the material could be covered in a semester. Each class consisted of students some of whom were hearing the lectures for the first time, some the second, some the third, and some for the fourth time. The lectures were very tightly structured and changed minimally from year to year.

Upon completion of Dr. Thomson's course, a diploma was awarded to the student, and this was issued by the South Bend College of Optics. Thomson was also president of the Thomson Optical Company of South Bend, a company that sold optical equipment to those who had completed the course at the college or through correspondence and who were therefore ready to begin the practice of optometry.

Dr. H. A. Thomson was clearly a busy man. In addition to his work running both college and correspondence course and his work as president of the Thomson Optical Company, he wrote a monthly column entitled "Query Department" in the optical magazine, *The Optical Journal Supplement*. Readers were invited to send questions to Dr. Thomson and some of the questions and answers were published, although all questions were answered. The description of the Query Department indicates the way the column was run:

"In this department we will answer questions pertaining to practical or technical optical work of interest to our readers. Our subscribers are invited to use this department freely when in doubt or difficulty. When writing for advice upon difficult cases the following information should be given: 1st. Age of patient. 2nd. What glasses, if any, have been previously worn, and for how long. 3rd. Visual acuteness of each eye separately, with and without glasses. 4th. Method of examination used and particulars of the test. No questions will receive attention unless signed by the inquirer in his own name, not necessarily for publication but as evidence of good faith. Address all inquires to Query Department, Optical Journal Supplement, care Dr. H. A. Thomson, South Bend, Ind."

The correspondence course in optics consisted of twenty lessons, two of these being sent to the student each week for a ten week period. The lessons were typed, single spaced on both sides of 8½ x 11 sheets and were mailed in No. 10 manila envelopes that required one cent postage. The average lesson was seven typed pages (four sheets of paper) and included questions for the student to answer. Thus the envelope that arrived each week at the student's home contained two lessons on eight or nine sheets of 8½ x 11 paper.

Dr. Thomson instructed the student to answer all questions but he requested that the answers *not* be returned to him. Instead, with each envelope after the first, Dr. Thomson included a page or two of answers and "explanations" to the questions of the previous lessons. Thus, the second week, the student received lessons 3 and 4, along with the explanations of the questions accompanying lessons

1 and 2. The exception was the questions that accompanied lessons 18 and 20. These the student was to answer in writing and return to Dr. Thomson as the final examination. Thomson also requested that the final payment for the course accompany the answers to the questions in lessons 18 and 20 so that he could have diplomas made up for those who had completed the course satisfactorily!

Thomson points out that "In case any of your answers fail to reach the required average, I will go over them carefully and send you a personal letter explaining where you have made errors, and will submit other examinations in their place, and will give you whatever explanations are necessary in order to qualify you for the diploma."

The entire Thomson course in optics contained 323 questions, an average of 16 per lesson. In terms of pages, the course consisted of 180 pages, 140 of these being textual material (550 words to the page or 75,000 words of total text), eleven pages of questions and 20 pages of answers or explanations to previous questions.[6] Thus the sum total of optometric education in 1895 could be typed on both sides of 85 sheets of 8½ x 11 paper.

The topics covered in the twenty lessons give some idea of the scope of optometric practice at the time optometry first evolved. The first five chapters cover what Thomson called physical optics, and is really a combination of physical optics, geometric optics and some discussion of ophthalmic optics. The sixth chapter described the eye and its refraction. The seventh and eighth chapters dealt with accommodation and convergence respectively, while the ninth and tenth chapters dealt with objective methods and subjective methods of testing vision. The next four chapters dealt respectively with hypermetropia, myopia, astigmatism, and anisometropia. Presbyopia was described in part of the chapter on anisometropia. The fifteenth and sixteenth chapters dealt with practical optometry and included also a discussion of practice management. The seventeenth chapter dealt with retinoscopy, the eighteenth with lenses and the nineteenth with muscle insufficiencies. The final chapter included a very brief description of the most common eye diseases, and included the advice that patients with such diseases be referred to an oculist. Clearly, the scope of optometry at the beginning was refraction and the supplying of spectacles only.

The text for the course was *Hartridge on Refraction*. The student was instructed to purchase the book from his local bookseller, or he could purchase one from the college for $1.50 plus 10c postage. Dr. Thomson does not state which edition of *Hartridge* was used, but it was probably the seventh edition published in 1894.[7] Although *Hartridge* was the only recommended textbook, Dr. Thomson did suggest that the student would benefit from reading the few pages on the anatomy of the eye in *Gray's Anatomy*. He suggested that the student borrow a copy of *Gray's Anatomy* from a physician in his home town and read the appropriate section.

Along with the fifth lesson, the student received a self-addressed post card from the Thomson Optical Company of South Bend, Indiana (Dr. H. A. Thomson, President). The card was a request to have a catalogue of trial sets and optical instruments sent to the student.

The total curriculum for home study graduates of the South Bend College of Optics at the turn of the century ran for ten weeks. Each week, the student was required to read about 7500 words written by Dr. Thomson and to answer 30 to 35 questions. He was also required to read a section in *Hartridge* each week. Since *Hartridge* contained about half as many words as Dr. Thomson's course, this assignment was not too rigorous.

Thomson utilized an interesting (and previously much used) teaching technique. Whenever he had presented an important concept, he summarized it and recommended that the student copy the summary. He instructed the student to purchase a note-book and copy all of the appropriate statements in it. Throughout the course, 214 such statements appeared. The student who completed the course and followed instructions would have a notebook in which he had copied 214 summary paragraphs. Dr. Thomson advised the student to save this notebook for reference after he began practice, since it would be a valuable collection of rules for the practitioner to follow.

Dr. Thomson offered his students the opportunity of changing their method of learning. Any student who wished to transfer from the correspondence course to the "attendant" course offered at the college could do so and the $25 that he had spent for the correspondence course would be applied toward the $50 tuition for the course in residence. If the student preferred to have his twenty correspondence lessons in bound book form, he could purchase such a book by sending Dr. Thomson $1.50 and returning the loose-leaf lessons.

Dr. Thomson's Correspondence Course in Optics gives the present day optometrist an idea of the scope of optometry at its beginning, and a look at early education. Today's optometrist is graduated from a college or university after a minimum of six years of academic training including lectures, laboratories and clinics. He has spent a year examining patients and practicing optometry in the college clinics.[8] His predecessor, however, the optometrist at the turn of the century, began practice after having read *Hartridge,* Dr. Thomson's 75,000 words, having copied the 214 important paragraphs in a notebook, and after having answered about 300 questions posed by Dr. Thomson. He was also probably armed with a trial lens set that he had bought from the Thomson Optical Company.

Although there is a tremendous difference between the early optometric courses like that of Dr. Thomson and the present day sophisticated optometric curriculum, the early courses served a very useful purpose. At the time when persons to test vision did not exist in nearly sufficient numbers, courses like Dr. Thomson's trained thousands of opticians to meet the public's need for vision care. Since the Thomson course covered only a fraction of the material learned by the present day optometric student, the practitioner of the time practiced only a small part of what today comprises optometry. The Thomson course differs from the modern optometric curriculum in the same way that a "refraction" differs from "complete scope optometric service."

Literature in the 1890's.

The series of 20 lessons used in the South Bend College of Optics and in the Thomson Correspondence Course in Optics were written by Dr. Thomson and copyrighted by him in 1895. The student was also required to read appropriate sections in *Hartridge on Refraction.* Other teachers who gave brief courses in vision testing at about this time also produced their own teaching materials. There were, however, books on sight testing in existence, and it is interesting that those offering courses found it necessary to produce their own materials. In the present section we shall review several of the books in the English language that were available in the 1890's to an optician or oculist who wished to learn how to test vision and prescribe spectacles.

The classical volume by Donders, *On the Anomalies of Accommodation and Refraction of the Eye*, was published in English in 1864.[9] Although Donders was Dutch and wrote in his native tongue, the book was translated from the author's manuscript by William Daniel Moore and appeared initially in English, published by the New Sydenham Society of London. Donders stated in the preface that it was his object "to make the book—notwithstanding its great size, useful and, in all its parts, easily accessible to the practical physician." His obvious success in placing the science of vision testing on a sound basis earned for him the name "Father of Modern Refraction."

Donders understood and explained the refractive anomalies, hypermetropia, myopia and astigmatism; he explained the accommodative mechanism and presbyopia; he discussed the relationship between accommodation and convergence and explained anomalies of binocular coordination. Donders' book had numerous case histories in it to increase its usefulness for the "practical" reader.

Although the material covered by Donders would have been of value to anyone wishing to test vision, and although it is clearly a work that placed "refraction" on a sound scientific basis, its size and complexity probably kept teachers like Thomson from adopting it as a teaching tool. Donders' book is certainly not the reading material that one would use in a one or two week course. It is probable that Donders' book was read by the teachers of the brief courses but was not required reading for students.

While Donders' book was designed for the practitioner, the scientific basis for much of vision testing appeared in book form almost simultaneously with the Donders book. The three volume textbook of Physiological Optics by Helmholtz also was published in the 1860's. This book, in German, was to go through two revisions and expansions before the third edition was translated into English by Southall in 1924. It is easily understood why teachers like Thomson did not recommend Helmholtz to the students. It was not available in English, it was designed to be a definitive discourse on the basic science of physiological optics rather than a book for the practitioner, and it was far too complex and complete a treatise for the brief courses offered in the United States in the 1890's.

In 1886, *Refraction and Accommodation of the Eye and Their Anomalies*, by E. Landolt of Paris appeared in English.[10] This book was published in Edinburgh, Scotland, and was translated under the author's supervision by C. M. Culver of Albany, New York. The Landolt book is about the same size as Donders, and is an update of Donder's similarly titled book. The book is divided into three portions: the first, a "Physical Portion," is a discourse on optics and lenses; the second section, the "Theoretical Portion," is devoted to the dioptric apparatus of the eye, the anomalies of refraction, and a strong section on optometers, ophthalmoscopes and other instruments useful in determining the refraction and accommodation of the eye; the third section, almost half of the total pages, the "Clinical Portion," is a treatise on the clinical practice of vision testing. Landolt in this section discusses the effect of lenses, the nature of refractive anomalies, and even has a section on "Orthoptic Exercises" using a stereoscope, and recommended by Landolt.

While the Landolt book, like Donders, is a complete work for the practitioner who would test vision and prescribe lenses, it was probably too complete for the brief courses offered in the United States in the 1890's. Landolt, like Donders, exhibits remarkable clinical wisdom; the present day optometrist is impressed that these two books, one over a hundred years old, the other over 80 years old, were so advanced for their time. The present day optometric curriculum neglects no topic covered by Donders or Landolt; but in the 1890's the teaching of vision testing was much too brief to allow the student to wend his way through these two "big" books.

While the books by Donders and Landolt were the two major texts on refractive anomalies, accommodation, and methods of measurement in the last half of the nineteenth century, these topics were also covered by several other authors. Some authors who wrote standard textbooks of ophthalmology included the topics of sight testing and prescribing spectacles as well as diseases of the eye. When one examines the general textbooks of ophthalmic medicine (ophthalmology) he immediately recognizes the influence of Donders. Authors of texts on diseases of the eye, prior to Donders, placed the responsibility for treating refractive anomalies and choosing spectacles on the patient and the optician but not on the oculist. Shortly after Donders' book appeared, however, the scope of eye medicine was broadened to include testing for refractive errors and specifying spectacles for them.

Jones[11] in 1847 wrote:

"But when a person finds it necessary to have recourse to glasses for shortsightedness, he should go to an optician, and select two or three pairs which appear to assist his vision best . . . and try them leisurely at home for a day or two before fixing his choice on one particular pair."

Jones offers the identical advice for farsightedness, i.e., visit an optician, choose two or three pairs of spectacles, and wear these a few days at home before choosing one of them.

Lawrence[12] in 1854 offered similar advice. He wrote: "When a nearsighted person wishes to be fitted with concave lenses, the simplest and surest plan is to try a series of them, at an optician's shop."

Lawrence also repeats the admonition of the ophthalmologist Mackenzie that if a patient wears concave lenses, "the disease (myopia) becomes not only confirmed but sometimes greatly aggravated."

The books by Jones and by Lawrence, both British ophthalmic surgeons, antedate Donders, and clearly relegate refractive anomalies and their correction by spectacles to the patient himself and to the optician. Two books that appeared in 1869, only 15 years after Lawrence and 5 years after Donders, offer a very different approach and clearly place the prescription of spectacles in the office of the eye physician rather than with the patient or the optician.

Wells,[13] a British ophthalmic surgeon, devotes much more space in his general textbook of ophthalmology to refractive errors and spectacles than did Lawrence or Jones. Wells urges physicians to learn the necessary optics and to test patients for appropriate spectacles. After discussing the optics of refraction, the anomalies of refraction (myopia, hypermetropia, astigmatism and presbyopia), Wells writes:

"From the perusal of the different anomalies of refraction and accommodation, the reader will have been sufficiently impressed with the importance of the proper and scientific selection of spectacles. I have no hesitation in saying that the empirical, haphazard plan of selection generally employed by opticians, is but too frequently attended by the worst consequences; and that eyes are often permanently injured, which might, by skillful treatment, have been preserved for years. For this reason, I must strongly urge upon medical men the necessity of not only examining the state of the eyes, and ascertaining the exact nature of the affection of refraction or accommodation, but of going even a step further than this, and determining with care and accuracy the number of the required lens. For this purpose they must possess a case of trial-glasses, containing a complete assortment of concave and convex lenses, glasses of corresponding number being kept by the optician. Written directions as to the focal distance or for reading, are to be sent to the optician."

Lawson,[14] a British ophthalmic surgeon whose textbook was also published in 1869, quotes from Donders and recommends that the eye physician use trial lenses to select the proper spectacles for the patient. Donders' work apparently was adopted by ophthalmological authors very rapidly. The publication of Donders in England and in English undoubtedly contributed to the short time span before the book's suggestions were adopted.

All major textbooks of ophthalmology or eye medicine from 1870 onward devote a section to refractive and accommodative anomalies and to the testing of vision for the prescription of spectacles. Instructions for testing vision using the trial case are included in each of these books. In the 25 years between 1870 and 1895 when Dr. Thomson wrote his course, several large textbooks of ophthalmology or diseases of the eye appeared. Each of these books devoted a section or two to a discussion of anomalies of refraction and accommodation, and to their correction by spectacles for which the physician was instructed to test. Among these general texts of ophthalmology appearing between the time of Donders and of Thomson was one by Angell[15] of Boston in 1873, by Buffum[16] of Chicago in 1884, by Nettleship[17] of Moorfields in London in 1890, and by Noyes[18] of New York in 1890.

During the period between Donders and Thomson, three major textbooks of ophthalmology went through several editions. These major texts by Fuchs of Germany,[19] DeSchweinitz of Philadelphia,[20] and Swanzy of Dublin, Ireland[21] all dealt with eye medicine and diseases of the eye; all included sections on the nature of and the testing for refractive anomalies and the use of spectacles for them.

The topic of refractive anomalies and their correction did not appear only in general textbooks of diseases of the eye or ophthalmology. During the last quarter of the 19th century several oculists authored small handbooks or teaching texts on refraction. These books were usually considerably briefer than Donders or Landolt. They were usually written by faculty members at various medical colleges or hospitals in the United States and Great Britain. They often took the form of handbooks. These books usually had a chapter or two on basic optics particularly the optics of spectacles lenses, chapters on myopia, hypermetropia, astigmatism, accommodation and presbyopia, methods of testing vision and measuring refractive errors, and a brief section on anomalies of binocular vision. Three books appeared between 1875 and 1895 and were available to Thomson at the time he was preparing his series of lessons.

Fenner, a physician in Louisville, Kentucky, wrote a book entitled "Vision: Its Optical Defects and the Adaptation of Spectacles," in 1875.[22] The author states that the book was intended for "the student, the physician, and to those of the general public who desire to obtain an insight into this department of science." Although this book had the usual chapters on optics, refractive anomalies and spectacles, it was not intended primarily as a text for oculists or opticians.

In 1877, Robert Brudenell Carter, an ophthalmic surgeon in London, published a brief book entitled "On Defects of Vision Which Are Remediable by Optical Appliances."[23] The text is based upon a series of lectures that Carter had delivered at the Royal College of Surgeons. Although Carter did not present material on the actual testing of vision or fitting of spectacles, he discussed the various refractive conditions and the spectacles that he would prescribe.

"The Refraction of the Eye" by Gustavus Hartridge,[24] an ophthalmic surgeon in London, was described by the author as "A Manual for Students." The first edition appeared in 1884 and a new edition appeared every year or two. In later editions, this classic became known as "Hartridge on Refraction." By the time the sixteenth edition had appeared in 1919, 38,000 copies had been printed.

The Hartridge book was organized so as to make it an ideal handbook for students. The dozen chapters are quite brief but give the student the material he will need to engage in vision testing and prescribing spectacles. The first chapter is a review of optics, and the second describes the refraction of the eye. The next three chapters describe methods of testing the refraction; the next five chapters deal respectively with hypermetropia, myopia, astigmatism, presbyopia and strabismus. The eleventh chapter is on asthenopia, and the last chapter discusses spectacles. A series of case reports is appended as are sample test types.

The earlier editions of Hartridge were published in England by J. & A. Churchill; the later editions in the United States by P. Blakiston's Sons and Co. In 1889, Francis Valk, an oculist in New York and faculty member at the New York Post-Graduate Medical School, published a series of his lectures[25] that covered much the same material as Hartridge. This book, like Hartridge, was obviously popular, for by 1905 it had already gone through four editions.

Clearly, when Dr. Thomson chose a textbook to accompany his set of lectures there was no dearth of books from which to choose. In choosing Hartridge, he picked the book that had the simplest writing, and complete coverage of the subject in the smallest number of words.

That the Thomson course was prepared at a period when there was great interest in the topic of vision testing is demonstrated by the fact that within a period of four years (1899–1903) at least six more books on refraction appeared in the English language. Each was written by a physician (three in the United States, and three in England) and each covered the same material as Valk or Hartridge had covered. Each was a small book and was intended for students who were learning to test vision and prescribe spectacles for refractive errors. For the most part, the format was quite similar for each book—a brief review of optics, a discussion of the errors of refraction and of methods of testing refraction, some discussion of binocular vision and a discussion of spectacles. These books, of course, were not available to Thomson when he prepared his lectures but were available during much of the period that the Thomson course was in use.

The Refractive and Ophthalmic Catechism by Lawrence J. Dailey[26] of New York appeared in 1898 and was described as being for the use of "General Practitioners, Opticians and Students." *The Handbook of Optics* by William Norwood Suter[27] of Washington, D.C. appeared in 1899 and was an attempt to give the student of ophthalmology a brief discourse on the optics of lenses and of refractive errors and of the instruments used in testing refraction of the eye. In 1899 the first edition of *Refraction and How to Refract*, a book that was to rival Hartridge in popularity, was published by James Thorington,[28] a professor at the Philadelphia Polyclinic and College for Graduates in Medicine. In 1901, J. Herbert Parsons of the Royal London (Moorfields) Ophthalmic Hospital published a little book[29] on ophthalmic optics including sections on refractive anomalies and the optics of testing equipment (ophthalmoscopy and retinoscopy). In 1903, Ernest Clarke of the same institution as Parsons in England published a handbook for students bearing the title of *The Errors of Accommodation and Refraction of the Eye and Their Treatment.*"[30] This book covered essentially the same material as Hartridge, Valk and Thorington. In the same year (1903), Campbell[31] also of London published a handbook entitled *The Refraction of the Eye and the Anomalies of the Ocular Muscles* that followed the same format—a section on optics, one on refraction of the eye, one on the instrument techniques for testing refraction of the eye, one on each of the refractive errors, one on spectacles, and one on binocular anomalies.

Each of these handbooks was a brief statement of the material covered earlier by Donders and by Landolt—much condensed and brought up to date. The large number of handbooks that appeared in the 1890's indicate the wide interest in the topic that must have existed at that time.

In reviewing the literature of the half century from 1860–1910, one is struck by the fact that almost all books were written by physicians. The major texts on refractive anomalies and their measurement by Donders and Landolt, the standard texts on ophthalmology which included refraction, and the large number of handbooks designed specifically for the student who would test vision and prescribe spectacles, were all written by physicians. Opticians had been learning sight-testing through apprenticeship, through work with patients for whom they made spectacles, and through personally directed study; but there was no literature. Some of the books, like Dailey's Catechism, were intended for both oculists and opticians, but all were written by physicians. Even the courses for opticians like that of Dr. Thomson (or McFatridge or Ketchum or Ring or Ruddy) were given to opticians by physicians.

Two other books of the period deserve comment, since both were intended for opticians. One was by the physician C. H. Brown[32] of Philadelphia, was entitled *The Optician's Manual* and was published in 1890; the other by William Bohne[33] called *Handbook for Opticians* appeared in its first edition in 1888 and is unique in that it is the only book for opticians written by an optician.

The Keystone, a magazine described as the *Organ of the Jewelry and Optical Trades*, was published in Philadelphia by Keystone Press. In each issue from May, 1890 to November, 1896 a series of articles on opticianry authored by C. H. Brown, M.D. appeared. Dr. Brown's column was titled "The Optician's Manual." Ultimately, these articles were published in two volumes as *The Optician's*

Manual, subtitled "A Treatise on the Science and Practice of Optics." The first volume contained chapters on optics, anatomy of the eye, lenses, the eye as an optical device, the use and value of glasses, instrumentation, methods of examining the eye, and presbyopia. The second volume, called the *Supplement to the Optician's Manual*, dealt primarily with myopia and hypermetropia. The first volume, over 400 pages, sold for $2.00; the supplement, over 200 pages, sold for $1.00.

The two volumes by Brown, appearing in the last decade of the 19th century, made a reasonably complete treatise on the material covered by Thomson in his course. The articles and the bound copies of the Manual were clearly intended for opticians. The author states in the preface to the first edition that, although the material has already been read by most opticians in the monthly magazine, it is published as a hard cover book in response to the demands of the opticians to serve as a reference book.

The similarity between Drs. Brown and Thomson is worth noting. Both were physicians, each conducted a monthly column in a magazine designed for opticians, and each produced material for the training of opticians in vision testing—Dr. Brown a pair of books and Dr. Thomson a correspondence course and a brief residence course.

All of the books reviewed thus far in the present section were written by physicians. Three contributions of opticians in this same period should be mentioned.

J. M. Johnston, born in 1844 in western New York, was trained originally for the church but in 1880 entered the Johnston Optical Company. In 1886 he published the *Eye Echo*, the first journal in America devoted exclusively to ophthalmic optics. In 1891 the name of the journal was changed to the *Eye Light*. In 1892 Johnston published "Eye Studies," a series of lessons on vision and visual tests, and in 1895 he started a school of optics including a correspondence course. The school and the correspondence course were based upon his series of lessons. His educational process, a journal, a series of lessons, a school, a correspondence course and an optical company, is all very similar to Dr. Thomson's schema.

W. Bohne, an optician in New Orleans, published a book in 1888 entitled *Hand-Book for Opticians*. The book was published by the author, and seemingly enjoyed a good sale for it went through three editions, the third edition appearing in 1895. Bohne's preface to the third edition gives a good picture of the status of opticianry in 1895:

> "The great progress our trade has made within the last five years is due to the able teachings of Optical Schools, and also to the increased study of the various books of instruction, lately published, which have enabled the workmen to follow that part of their vocation, which comprises the selection of spectacles in a more scientific way than formerly, when each optician had to commence for

himself at the bottom of his trade, and only by incessant exertion gradually
reached the required proficiency.

. . . . Most of these books are written to assist the oculist, and only secondarily
the optician, in the selection and adaptation of spectacles."

Bohne mentions the handbooks of Hartridge, Valk, Tiffany, and notes that
his book is not as good on the sections on refractive errors (myopia, hypermetropia, astigmatism, and presbyopia) but that it does deal with "the technicalities
of the trade" which the others do not. He urges his readers to consult the handbooks written primarily for the oculist in order to obtain an understanding of
anomalies of refraction and accommodation.

Bohne's book demonstrates clearly the role of the optician in the 1890's. He
gives brief biographies of the famous opticians (including his own) and one is
struck by the number whose "fame" rested upon work with telescopes and microscopes and lenses in general, and how few owed their renown to spectacles.
In the section of his book on Miscellanies, Bohne describes his concept of the
relationship that opticians and oculists should bear to each other:

Oculist and Optician.—"Where does the province of the oculist end and that of
the optician begin?" This question is most essential, in order to establish a
sound *modus vivendi* between the parties whose vocations are so closely related
as those of the optician and oculist.

To answer such a question we must be guided by the most scrupulous sense of
equity, even at the risk of dampening the ambitious ardor of some enthusiasts
on either side; otherwise we may be accused of partiality and unfairness. The
present position of oculists versus opticians is that of two competitors, each of
whom is claiming the lion's share of the spectacle trade; let us see by what
right.—Opticians, as the manufacturers of spectacles, have been for many years
the exclusive dispensers of their goods, and a good many of them did acquire
great skill in fitting all cases of presbyopia, and most cases of myopia and
hypermetropia, although the latter was not yet known by that name; but it
was done after all in a hap-hazard way, and many cases were abandoned by
them as incurable. There was no optician, to my knowledge, who explored such
"incurable" cases, and tried to relieve those unfortunate sufferers, until some
oculists and physicists took them in hand, and succeeded, by the application of
mydriatics and the aid of the ophthalmoscope (also an invention of a
physician), to overcome their trouble by cylindric glasses; thus increasing
greatly the formerly restricted use of spectacles.

These facts could not have prevented us from appropriating inventions which
now belong to the world, if it were not for the protection of the public at large,
to confine the application of drugs to the medical department. In my opinion,
therefore, the line of the province of oculists should be drawn to such cases
where a *mydriatic has to be employed*. This leaves to us not only all cases we
formerly served, but adds to them many new ones. Self-interest and improper

ambition may overstep this integral limit of each legitimate province, but that cannot be avoided as long as human nature is so frail.

The oculist may find this line drawn a little too narrow, and may point to the many spectacle dealers who have hardly elevated themselves above the level of simple mechanics. But there are poor practitioners as well as experts in every occupation, not only among opticians.

If we take in consideration the close relationship of the two branches of practical optics from a *business standpoint*, we must admit that the efforts of the oculists to prescribe glasses have only increased our usefulness, and have elevated our insignificant occupation as simple spectacle vendors to a scientific trade, which to-day embraces numerous investigators and able writers. We have, therefore, no reason to be jealous of their success, which benefits us materially as well as intellectually.

In the 1890's many opticians felt that the testing of vision was not the province of the optician. Bohne, although he does teach his reader to test vision, seems to fall within this category. Bohne believed that only the simplest refractive errors could be measured by opticians. He wrote:

". . . . there are cases beyond the sphere of opticians, *i.e.* when it is impossible to make the right diagnosis without preparing the eye for such an examination. These patients should be turned over to an oculist; it would be an act of "charlatanry" on our part to pretend to do full justice to such cases. Confine your skill to the limits of your trade, and you will be convinced that it requires all your knowledge, intelligence and energy to fill the place of an expert optician. Over-ambitious young men may commit the error of trying to combine the two branches of an oculist and an optician as far as spectacles are concerned; but is it not the mistake of a builder who would be his own architect, the apothecary his own doctor? The public in general fares better if these branches are divided, and ably represented by competent specialists; on one side the scientific oculist, on the other side the skillful optician, both experts in their particular branches. If we play oculist, why should not the oculist play optician, and keep a stock of spectacles on hand? Therefore my advice, *"Suum ciuque."*

Charles F. Prentice, to whom the title "Father of Optometry" has been given, was a practicing optician in New York beginning in 1878. Well educated in optics in Germany, Prentice published several scientific papers on optical problems of lenses, many of them in ophthalmological journals. Unlike Bohne, Prentice believed that he had sufficient knowledge to test vision for spectacles. Disagreement with a physician, who did not question an optician's right to test vision but who maintained that if he charged for this service he was setting himself up as an oculist, brought Prentice into leadership in the movement for legal recognition of optometry.

Bohne and Prentice were the two opticians whose writings in the period prior to 1900 were of significance—Bohne as a writer of a handbook for opticians but with a philosophy of opticians only testing for spectacles in the simplest cases, and Prentice as a recognized optical scientist.

As one reviews the books of the period prior to 1900, he wonders at the need for series of lessons like those of Thomson. There were several regular textbooks that contained the same material. The Thomson course (and the several others like it that appeared) was more than a textbook. It was, essentially, a system of programmed learning—textual material, questions and answers, important statements to be copied, explanations of the answers. The Thomson course and others like it were the means whereby oculists and opticians could learn enough about vision testing so that they could practice this art. The course was a needed step between the period of Donders, a period of discovery, and the time that college courses were established to teach vision testing.

Changes in Scope of Optometric Practice—1890's to Present.

The first optometrists were opticians who began testing vision so that they could supply spectacles specifically designed for the needs of an individual patient. The scope of optometric practice in the 1890's was simply the testing of vision and the supplying of spectacles.

During the first half of the twentieth century, as optometry attained legislative recognition, an educational system and professional organizations, the scope of practice changed markedly. The scope broadened as new areas were added to the practice of optometry.

One of the first areas of broadened scope that optometrists added was the responsibility for the recognition of diseases of the eye. A change of philosophy came about as well as an increased utilization of new techniques for pathology recognition. The first optician-optometrists regarded their function as providing spectacles for patients with healthy eyes. Therefore they regarded any observation of a patient for disease as being necessary to *limit* the patients whom they fitted with spectacles to those who had healthy eyes. The earliest optometrists recognized disease so that they would know which patients *not* to fit with spectacles. But as patients began consulting optometrists as primary health practitioners, the optometrists recognized that they had a greater responsibility to the patient with ocular disease or with general disease that manifested itself in the eyes, than merely to refuse to supply him with spectacles. If optometrists were to do the best they could for patients it was not enough to limit their services to those with healthy eyes. The optometrist had a responsibility to recognize ocular and general disease *and* to advise the patient of what steps he should take next. Optometrists began to use the ophthalmoscope, the tangent screen, the tonometer, and the biomicroscope—not to limit the sale of spectacles to those with healthy eyes but to serve properly those who had eye and general disease. The optometrist today tries to recognize glaucoma in its earliest stages so that he can refer the patient for medical consultation. Whether or not he supplies spectacles for the patient's vision is immaterial; as a primary health care provider, the optometrist must be able to recognize many diseases that manifest themselves in the eye so that he can move the patient along to the next needed health service.

A second area of broadened scope was in the treatment of anomalies of binocular vision through lenses (prisms), and through rehabilitative visual training or orthoptics. Optometrists recognized that many patients could be benefitted through training and educative procedures that would enable the patient to use his vision more comfortably and more effectively. Thus, optometrists began not only to supply spectacles but to work with patients in the rehabilitation of neuromuscular binocular abnormalities through vision training.

A third area of broadened scope occurred when optometrists recognized that patients required not only spectacles, but advice on vision. If a patient was using improper illumination, spectacles alone would not solve his visual problem. If a patient's occupation presented special visual requirements the patient required lenses for specific tasks *and* advice on how to use his eyes and spectacles on his job. Thus, the optometrist became a health care provider who advised patients on ocular hygiene, illumination, occupational vision and similar topics.

During the first half of the twentieth century, several new or special types of lenses were developed. The scope of optometric practice broadened to include the testing for and supplying of aniseikonic lenses, contact lenses and low vision aids to magnify objects and enable persons with reduced vision to attain useful vision. Each of these new devices broadened the scope of optometric practice. To supply contact lenses one must concern himself with the physiology of the cornea, a topic of little importance in supplying spectacle lenses. To supply a low vision aid often requires deep understanding of the psychology of the partially-sighted patient as well as of the optics of magnification systems. As new optical devices and lenses were developed, the scope of optometric practice was broadened to include not only the device but all of the basic knowledge required to supply the device with optimal results.

During the first half of the twentieth century, the optometric practice developed into the general practice of eye and vision care. Optometric scope did *not* include medical or surgical care of the eyes. This always was and remained the practice of medicine. But optometric scope included all other aspects of vision care. The scope of ophthalmology was everything that an optometrist did plus eye medicine and surgery. In the large cities of the United States there was usually a heavy concentration of eye physicians, and the role of optometrists was not important. But the number of optometrists from almost the beginning was far greater than the number of eye physicians, and optometrists often chose the smaller cities and towns as locations for their practices. Because the United States is so large geographically, and because the number of optometrists was not large and many chose the smaller communities, many communities were served only by one optometrist. These optometrists, like the practitioners of general medicine in the smaller communities, were called upon to care for whatever problems fell within their scope and to refer to specialists in neighboring larger cities those patients who required skills beyond their scope. Due to the need of the public, the optometrist developed into the general practitioner in the eye care field.

Today, optometry is the third largest primary health care profession in the United States. Optometry often serves as the entry point of the patient into the health care system. A patient, for example, with eye symptoms of a general disease may often seek the optometrist and he is then referred by the optometrist to an appropriate medical practitioner.

The optometrist evolved from the optician, a maker and supplier of spectacles. In the beginning he was an optician who had learned to test vision so that the spectacles he supplied were designed for the individual patient. As new unmet needs of the public were recognized, the optometrist increased his scope of practice and simultaneously added appropriate new material to the curriculum of optometric educational institutions. Ultimately the optometrist developed into the general practitioner in the eye care field—the role he plays in health care in the United States today.

The Thomson Correspondence Course in Optics is significant in the history of optometry because it is an early addition of knowledge to meet a need of the public. The Thomson course is the material that an optician added to his education in order to enable him to enlarge his scope to include testing individual patients for spectacles. It is the first instance of the mechanism through which optometry developed into an important health care profession—namely by recognizing a need of the public and obtaining the education necessary to meet the need. This same pattern was to occur again and again, and it is noteworthy that the pattern was established at the very beginning of optometry's modern history.

Summary

By 1890, due to advances in lens making made by opticians, physicists and other scientists, it was possible to design a lens for an individual that had spherical, cylindrical and prismatic power and it was also possible to construct a bifocal lens that had two separate foci and mount this in a single spectacle frame. The craft of opticianry had become sufficiently sophisticated so that prefabricated spectacles were no longer desirable and it was possible to make a pair of spectacles that were suited to one (and only one) individual patient. It was necessary if one were to give the best vision care to test the vision and make spectacles for the individual patient. Some opticians, like the Prentices of New York City or the McAllisters of Philadelphia, had learned to test vision and were offering this service to patients. Other opticians, however, argued that vision testing was beyond the scope of opticianry. Thus, two groups of opticians existed.[34]

By 1890, instruments for testing vision and testing techniques had been developed, mainly by those who followed the teachings of Donders. Among the medical eye practitioners or oculists, there was also a lack of agreement on what the scope of medical eye practice was. Some oculists tested vision and wrote a formula for spectacles to be supplied by an optician; others, however, still influenced by an earlier aversion to spectacles or recognizing their own lack of training in vision testing, did not test vision for spectacles.

In the 1890's there was no legal constraint against anyone examining vision. Anyone who felt he was capable of testing vision and supplying spectacles was able to do so.

Clearly, since neither opticians nor oculists had been trained to test vision, and since there were no legal requirements for the education one needed to test vision, and since some members of each group wished to test vision, there would be a great demand for training in vision testing. This demand by both opticians and oculists explains the large number of short courses both in-residence and correspondence that sprang up. Some oculists who had studied Donders and had mastered enough optics to understand vision testing, often became the teachers in the brief courses that were offered. The demand by both opticians and oculists also explains why many of the early schools or courses accepted opticians and oculists in the same courses on sight testing. It was to meet the demand for knowledge about vision testing that courses like Dr. Thomson's Correspondence Course were prepared, and offered.

By the end of the first decade of the twentieth century, the situation had changed sufficiently to make the short courses no longer needed. Several states had adopted optometry laws, setting forth the educational requirements for those who would test vision. Oculists and all physicians were exempt from these requirements since the vision testing that they did was considered to be a part of their medical practice. The opticians who tested vision separated from those who wished to supply spectacles only. These vision testing opticians became the first optometrists and began attaining the milestones that characterize a profession in the United States. They established an education system, obtained licensing legislation, and formed professional associations.

The need for brief courses in optics existed for only a very brief period. Courses like that of Dr. Thomson had life spans of less than 20 years. 1890 to 1910 was a period when the need for a large number of professionals who would test vision was recognized by opticians and oculists who could see what the future public needs would be. Opticians needed such courses until the early 1900's when regular optometric colleges were founded. Oculists needed such courses until the teaching of sight testing became a part of the regular training program for eye physicians. By 1910, both optometrists and oculists were learning sight testing in regular training institutions of their respective professions. But between 1890 and 1910, thousands of oculists and opticians who were *already in practice*, whose formal training had been completed, had to be taught optometry. It was to fill this need that courses like that of Thomson were designed.

The importance of the Thomson course and others like it in history is two-fold. First, it tells us the state of knowledge in "optometry" at about the time the move toward a new profession in the United States began. Second, it is an example of a course designed to help educate opticians and oculists in "optometry" during a period between the time of discovery of new material and the time when regular educational systems would take over.

Comparison of the Thomson course with his present scope and knowledge will give the modern optometrist a feeling for what advances have been made during the 75 years of optometry's development.

REFERENCES

1. At the turn of the century the word optometrist to describe one who examined eyes and prescribed lenses was not universally accepted. Charles Prentice, "father of the profession," preferred the word opticist, and described himself as an opticist. The first optometric association was named the American Association of Opticians, and although this association endorsed the title "optometrist" in 1903, the title of the organization was not changed to the American Optical Association until 1910 and the word "optometry" did not appear in the name of the organization until 1918. The first State law, that of Minnesota, did use the terms "optometry" and "optometrist" in 1901. As the scope of optometry expanded over the years it turned out that the term "optometry," implying physical measurement as it does, was a poor choice, but this name remained. In England, the name for the group of opticians who took on the function of testing vision was "ophthalmic opticians," and this is probably a better term, although the term of Prentice, "opticist," was probably the best of those used.

2. The basic science or pre-optometry courses can be completed in two years. However, more than half of the students who enter optometry school have completed three or four years as undergraduates. Six years of college work, therefore, is the minimum but more than half of today's optometry students have spent seven or eight years after high school in studying to become optometrists.

3. Optometric Education: A summary report—National Study of Optometric Education. Robert J. Havighurst, Study Director. National Commission on Accrediting, Washington, D.C., March, 1973.

4. Borish, Irvin M. Clinical Refraction. Third Edition, Chicago, The Professional Press Inc., 1970.

5. This early method of mass-producing spectacles and allowing the customer to choose for himself the pair that seems most suitable is still used in those of the United States that allow spectacles to be sold over-the-counter by variety stores or pharmacies.

6. About nine of the pages were blank, being the reverse side of material requiring one page only.

7. There were several books that Dr. Thomson could have chosen for the textbook in his course. The texts that were available during the last decade of the nineteenth century will be discussed in the next section of this introductory chapter.

8. For a fuller discussion of the history of optometric educational institutions, the reader is referred to The Optometric Profession by Monroe J. Hirsch and Ralph E. Wick, Philadelphia, Chilton Book Company, 1968.

9. Donders, F. C. On the Anomalies of Accommodation and Refraction of the Eye. London, The New Sydenham Society, 1864.

10. Landolt, E. The Refraction and Accommodation of the Eye and Their Anomalies. Edinburgh, Young J. Pentland, 1886.

11. Jones, T. Wharton. The Principles and Practice of Ophthalmic Medicine and Surgery. Edited by Isaac Hays. American Edition. Philadelphia, Lea and Blanchard, 1847.

12. Lawrence, W. A. Treatise on Diseases of the Eye. Edited by Isaac Hays. American Edition. Philadelphia, Lea and Blanchard, 1854.

13. Wells, J. Soelberg. A Treatise on the Diseases of the Eye. American Edition. Philadelphia, Henry C. Lea, 1869.

14. Lawson, George. Diseases and Injuries of the Eye. Philadelphia, Lindsay and Blakiston, 1869.

15. Angell, Henry C. A Treatise on Diseases of the Eye. Boston, James Campbell, 1873.

16. Buffum, J. H. The Diseases of the Eye. Chicago, Gross and Delbridge, 1884.

17. Nettleship, Edward. Diseases of the Eye. Philadelphia, Lea Brothers and Co., 1890.

18. Noyes, Henry D. A Text-book of Diseases of the Eye. New York, William Wood and Co., 1890.

19. Fuchs, Ernest (translated by Alexander Duane). Textbook of Ophthalmology.

20. DeSchweinitz, George C. Diseases of the Eye.

21. Swanzy, Henry R. Diseases of the Eye.

22. Fenner, C. S. Vision: Its Optical Defects, and the Adaptation of Spectacles. Philadelphia, Lindsay and Blakiston, 1875.

23. Carter, Robert Brundenell. On Defects of Vision which are Remediable by Optical Appliances. London, Macmillan and Co., 1877.

24. Hartridge, Gustavus. The Refraction of the Eye. London, J. & A. Churchill, 1884. (Later editions were published in the United States by P. Blakiston's Son & Co.)

25. Valk, Francis. Lectures on the Errors of Refraction and their Correction with Glasses. New York, G. P. Putnam's Sons, 1895.

26. Dailey, Lawrence J. Refractive and Ophthalmic Catechism. Gloverville, New York, Collins Publishing Co., 1898.

27. Suter, William Norwood. Handbook of Optics. New York, The Macmillan Company, 1899.

28. Thorington, James. Refraction and How to Refract. Philadelphia, P. Blakiston's Son & Co., 1899.

29. Parsons, J. Herbert. Elementary Ophthalmic Optics. London, J. & A. Churchill, 1901.

30. Clarke, Ernest. The Errors of Accommodation and Refraction of the Eye. New York, William Wood and Company, 1903.

31. Campbell, Kenneth. The Refraction of the Eye and the Anomalies of the Ocular Muscles. New York, William Wood and Company, 1903.

32. Brown, C. H. The Optician's Manual. Philadelphia, The Keystone (date of 1st edition was between 1890–1899).

33. Bohne, W. Handbook for Opticians. New Orleans, La., A. B. Griswold & Co., 1888.

34. In England, the same split occurred among opticians. Here, each group retained the name optician—those that did sight testing becoming known as ophthalmic opticians, the others dispensing opticians. The term optometrist was never adopted in England, and to this day the British counterpart of the American optometrist is the ophthalmic optician.

TABLE OF CONTENTS*

* This Table of Contents was not supplied by Dr. Thomson but was constructed by the editor of this volume to help the reader.

(The questions on Lessons No. 18 and No. 20 comprised the final examination in the Course)

DR. THOMSON'S 1895 CORRESPONDENCE COURSE

IN OPTICS.

South Bend, Ind.

To My Students:

I inclose you herewith Lessons No. 1 and 2. We will commence at the beginning and take up each subject in its regular order, so that not a single point may be missed. I shall endeavor in every way to make you thoroughly competent and would ask your co-operation in making the course everything we could desire. Do not hurry or skim over the work, but make it a point all through, never to leave a single subject until every phase of it is thoroughly understood from all sides. This is important, as the subjects will be presented in the order in which they will have the most bearing upon one another, and the loss of a single point will make all the succeeding lessons more difficult. In the lessons, as I leave one subject to take up another, I will make a dividing line like this:

————o◯o————

so when you come to such a line you may know that the subject is finished and another about to begin. Do not think of the lessons as a whole, but only consider one subject at a time and never mind the rest until that subject is perfectly mastered. By following this rule you will be surprised how rapidly you will advance and how thoroughly all the past subjects will be understood. It will be necessary that you have a text book and a note book. The text book which we shall follow is "Hartridge on Refraction." This will also make you a valuable hand book for daily use as long as you continue in the work. You can get it of any dealer, or I will be pleased to mail it to you on receipt of price, $1.50 and ten cents for postage. Any good blank book will do for a note book. In every lesson there will be notes and rules given for you to copy as you go along. Do not neglect to do this, and at the close of the course you will have a collection of valuable rules which will always be of service to you. Number them as you go, for we will refer to them by number from time to time. After you have finished a lesson to your satisfaction, take your note book and beginning at Rule No. 1, go over each one carefully and see that it is perfectly clear to you; if not, turn to that particular subject in the lesson and go over it again until it is thoroughly understood.

When this is done turn to the questions and see if you can answer each one to your satisfaction. I wish that every member of the class would not only try to answer them orally but would also write down the answers the best you can and place them on file for comparison and reference. I am going to send with the next lesson a list of correct answers to these questions together with an explanation upon each and it will be a great advantage to compare your own answers to these explanations and in that way find your weak points. I shall touch upon the errors that pupils are likely to make in answering them.

I know that you are in earnest in this work and that you want to get the very best possible good out of the course. If you will follow all of the instructions carefully and with the determination to make the course a success, I promise you I will not be behind in the effort. Everything will depend upon earnest and honest work on your part.

Do not send in your answers but hold them there to compare with the answers that I will send you next week. I will send answers and explanations each week upon the questions asked in the preceding lessons. At the close of the course I will send you a FINAL EXAMINATION bearing upon all of the subjects over which we have passed and this FINAL EXAMINATION you are to answer and send to me. Your percentage will be based upon your answers. If you reach the required average on each subject you will then be eligible to the diploma and degree. If you fall below on any subject I will give you additional instruction upon that subject until you have a thorough understanding of it.

If at any time during the course the answers and explanations upon any of the subjects are not sufficiently clear, you may feel at liberty to write and ask me questions concerning them.

At the end of each lesson I will designate certain pages in your text book which you will study between mails and which will be a necessary preparation for the next lesson. The first few lessons may, perhaps, be a little dry, but if you are patient and thorough in the work, we will soon be into the interesting portions.

Trusting that the course may prove both pleasant and profitable, I am,

Yours truly,

DR. H. A. THOMSON.

LESSON NO. 1.

General Optics.

As THE SCIENCE of Optics consists of the study of the laws of light it will be first in order to consider what light is.

If a pebble is dropped into a pond of water, there will be a circle of waves started from the point where the stone struck, which circle will continue to grow larger and larger until it has reached the limits of the pond.

If we strike our hands together there will be a disturbance created in the air similar to that which was created in the water by the stone striking it, and waves in the air will be formed which will travel in every direction in constantly increasing circles (or rather globes or spheres, for these waves travel up, down, and in every direction, while those on the water only travel laterally), until it has expended its power. These waves in the air are called "Sound Waves" and one of them dashing against the drum of the ear produces a sensation in the Auditory Nerve, which is transmitted to the brain and constitutes what we call sound.

In addition to water and air there exists a highly elastic, gaseous substance, which pervades all space throughout the universe, and is present even in the pores and between the atoms and particles of every substance. This gaseous substance is known as Luminiferous Aether, and a disturbance created within it is transmitted in every direction by means of waves similar to the sound waves of the air. A portion of these waves entering the eye and dashing against the retina produce a sensation in the Optic Nerve which being transmitted along that nerve to the brain, constitutes what we call Light. The atoms and particles of a luminous body are supposed to be in a constant state of very rapid vibration which motion is communicated to the Aether and then transmitted in all directions in spherical waves.

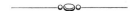

Light may come to us either from Luminous or Non-luminous Bodies. A Luminous Body is one in which light originates (as the Sun, a gas flame, etc.).

A Non-luminous Body does not originate light of itself, but may be rendered temporarily luminous by light from a luminous body being reflected from it. Thus the Moon is a Non-luminous body, but is made visible by the waves from the Sun falling upon it and being thrown off again in the direction of the Earth.

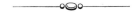

As we consider their waves in their movement, they may be divided into three classes, viz.: Rays, Pencils, Beams.

Head the first page of your notebook "Optics" and copy the following three notes, numbering them as you write:

1. A Ray is a single line of light.

2. A Pencil is a number of rays diverging from, or converging toward some point.

3. A Beam is a collection of rays all traveling parallel to each other.

The above definitions may be made more comprehensive by a glance at the following diagram.

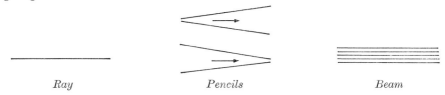

      Ray   *Pencils*   *Beam*

We have seen that light radiates from a luminous point in every direction, the spherical wave constantly increasing in size as it advances. Rays then, in leaving the luminous point must naturally be diverging. In fact all rays in nature are originally diverging, and in order to have parallel or converging rays, these diverging rays must first undergo a change of direction by artificial means.

Rays entering the eye from a given point will (as we have seen) be divergent, but the amount of the divergence will vary greatly as the point is moved nearer to, or farther from the eye. Thus by the following diagram we see that the rays in Fig. A, coming from a point quite near the eye, will enter the eye with considerable divergence. In Fig. B, the point having been removed farther from the eye, the rays are less di-

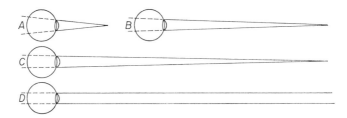

verging. Fig. C shows a still greater distance and still less divergence, while in Fig. D the point has been removed to a place so remote that the rays appear to the naked eye to be actually parallel. Rays coming from a distance of 6 meters (20 feet) or more are so near parallel that the eye is incapable of distinguishing the difference. In our studies therefore, we will hereafter consider all rays coming from a distance of 6 meters or beyond as parallel rays and a collection of these rays will, of course, constitute a beam (See Note 3). Copy in your notebook the following:

    4. The nearer the source of light to the eye the more divergent the rays.

    5. The more distant the light the less divergent the rays.

    6. If the light be removed to a distance of 6 meters (20 feet) or more the rays will enter the eye practically parallel.

In speaking of 20 feet or more we shall call the distance an "Infinite Distance" or "Infinity," and in speaking of a distance of less than 20 feet we shall call it a "Finite Distance." Thus the Sun, or the house across the street is at an Infinite Distance; the book which we hold in our hand is at a Finite Distance.

The rapidity of light is about 186,000 miles per second. In passing through dense substances, as air, water, glass, diamond, etc., the rapidity is lessened. Copy:

7. *The denser the substance through which light passes the less rapidly will it travel.*

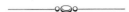

A ray of light traveling in any medium (or substance) will always travel in a straight line unless interrupted by coming in contact with some impediment or by leaving the first medium and entering another. Thus light moving through air will continue straight unless it comes in contact with some object, as a building, or a tree, in which case it will be thrown off in a new direction and will again continue straight until the next interruption; or, if the light enters another medium, as water, it may be changed in its course at the moment it enters the new medium, but after once getting fully into the new medium it will again proceed straight as before. Copy:

8. *Light always travels in straight lines so long as it continues uninterrupted in the same medium.*

The statement that light travels in straight lines may be proved by a number of very simple examples. For instance you have seen, hundreds of times, a ray of light entering through a small hole into a dark room, or building, and noticed the perfectly straight line of light passing from the hole to the floor where the rays struck. (N. B. You would not have been able to see this line at all had it not been for the particles of dust in the air which were illuminated by the passing light and some of the light thrown off in the direction of your eye). Another proof of the same statement may be shown by the following experiment: Take two cards of the size of postal cards or larger, and through the center of one make a small aperture about as large as the head of a pin.

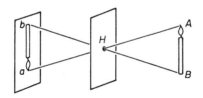

Now, if you will hold this card in front of a gas or lamp flame, and the other card still farther back the following will take place: Of all the rays which leave the point A, of the candle AB, only those going in the direction of the aperture H can pass through the card. If it be true that rays move in straight lines, the ray from A, after passing through the aperture H, must continue in the same direction as before, and will strike card 2 at "a." Rays from the point B will likewise pass through the aperture H and continuing in the same direction will strike card 2 at "b." The same will be true of all points situated between A and B, rays coming from them taking their places on card 2 between "b" and "a." Thus a perfect inverted picture of the candle AB will be produced upon card 2 at "ba." It must be clear that if light did not travel in straight lines this picture could not have been produced, but that the rays striking the card without regard to definite direction would only succeed in illuminating the card.

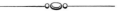

We have spoken of light coming in contact with different substances. Some of these substances are so constructed as to allow light to pass through them while others will not. If we consider them according to their various constructions, they may be divided into three classes: Transparent, Translucent, Opaque. Copy:

> *9. A Transparent Substance is one through which light readily passes (as glass, air, water).*

> *10. A Translucent Substance is one through which light will pass but so imperfectly that objects cannot be distinguished through them (as ground glass, horn).*

> *11. Opaque Substances are those which will not transmit light, (as wood, metals.)*

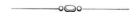

In order that we may be able to determine the SIZE and DISTANCE of any object, it is necessary that our eyes have some method of measurement by which they may assist us in our judgment of these two important elements. At what a loss we would be if it were impossible to say how far away some object might be, or, of what size. Fortunately we have a means of determining these questions and that means exists in what is known as the Visual Angle. Copy:

> *12. The Visual Angle is an angle formed by rays from the extreme points of an object, coming together at the center of the eye.*

Thus in the diagram the arrow AB, represents an object of a certain size at a cer-

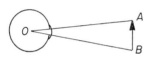
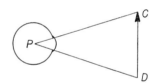

tain distance from the eye, and the arrow CD, represents another object of a larger size, but at the same distance from the eye. By drawing lines from A and B to the eye, the angle AOB will be the Visual Angle. Likewise lines drawn from C and D, to the eye will form the Visual Angle CPD. But the angle CPD is larger than the angle AOB. Hence the following rule. Copy:

> *13. For the same distance the Visual Angle increases with the size of the object.*

In the next diagram the arrow AB and CD represents two objects of the same size

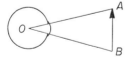
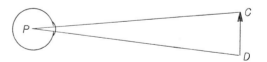

but at different distances from the eye. The Visual Angle CPD is smaller than the Visual Angle AOB. Hence the following rule. Copy:

> *14. For the same object the Visual Angle decreases with the distance of the object.*

A thorough understanding of the Visual Angle as given above is one of the most important and necessary parts of this entire lesson, as reference to the Visual Angle will be made in nearly every subsequent lesson. I would suggest, therefore, that you study the above explanations and rules very carefully, over and over again, until you are perfectly conversant with them.

———————o◯o———————

If a collection of rays come in contact with any substance a part of them will become annihilated, or destroyed. This always takes place regardless of the construction or material of the substance, although the number of rays destroyed varies with the different substances. This destroying or annihilating power is called "Absorption," of which we shall speak farther on. Another portion of the rays will be thrown back in a new direction and will proceed again in their new course. This power of throwing back waves of light is called "Reflection," which we shall also consider later. (A good illustration of the reflection of waves may be seen in a pail of water. If you suddenly jar the pail a circle of ripples or waves will start at the center and travel across the water to the sides, when it will be reflected, or thrown back again toward the center. This movement from the center to the sides and back to the center will continue until the force of the blow has expended itself.)

If our substance be a transparent one, still another effect is produced, viz.: a portion of the rays will pass through the substance and proceed on their way. This is called Transmission, and occurs in every Transparent or Translucent substance. Do not imagine as so many do, that all the rays pass through a transparent substance, for it is impossible to construct a substance so transparent that some of the rays will not be Absorbed and some Reflected.

Transmitted rays do not always pass through the transparent substance without changing their course, but may under certain conditions be bent into a new direction. This bending power is called "Refraction," a property with which we shall have considerable to do as we proceed in our studies.

Three things then may occur to light coming in contact with a substance, viz.: Absorption, Reflection and Transmission, and a portion of the transmitted rays, under certain conditions, may be Refracted. Copy:

15. *Light falling upon a substance may be Absorbed, Reflected, or Transmitted.*
16. *Transmitted light, if passed through any medium of different density than the one it previously left, MAY be Refracted.*

The science of Optics may therefore be classified under three heads, viz.: Absorption, Reflection (or Catoptrics) and Transmission. Under the latter head we will place Refraction (or Dioptrics.) Copy the following diagram in your notebook next after Rule 16.

Optics.
$\begin{cases} \textit{Absorption.} \\ \\ \textit{Reflection (or Catoptrics).} \\ \\ \textit{Transmission.} \end{cases}$ $\begin{cases} \textit{Refraction (or Dioptrics).} \end{cases}$

These subjects we will now take up in their regular oder, ending Lesson No. 1 with a consideration of Absorption.

Absorption.

Probably the best comparison I could make in illustrating this subject would be a row of piles, or stakes, driven along the edge of a lake to act as a breakwater. The waves dashing among these piles are so chopped and broken up that no trace of them remains. This same phenomena takes place in the Absorption of light. Even the most highly polished surface, if examined under a microscope, will show an infinite number of rough, uneven projections, sufficient to break up and destroy some of the light waves.

If a plate of glass is very thin, it will be almost perfectly transparent, but if the thickness is increased the transparency will be diminished, and it may be made of sufficient thickness to transmit no light at all. Each increase in thickness therefore, weakens the vibrations until at length the waves are utterly destroyed.

Even the purest air absorbs light so rapidly that the Sun's rays could not penetrate to the earth if the atmosphere had a depth of 700 miles. Gold, on the other hand, may be made so thin as to transmit light of a violet-green color.

Lesson No. 2 will take up the study of Reflection. In the meantime, after you have written your answers, and before beginning Lesson No. 2, I would advise a careful study of the first three pages of HARTRIDGE, ending at "Reflection by a Curved Surface" on the third page. You cannot study it too thoroughly.

(*End of Lesson No. 1.*)

QUESTIONS ON LESSON NO. 1.

1. Give your understanding of Light in twenty words or less.
2. How is the disturbance created from which light waves originate?
3. What is a body called which creates this disturbance?
4. Do we get light from any other bodies? If so, what?
5. Explain how light may come to us from such bodies.
6. Give examples.
7. What is Reflection?
8. Tell me in your own language all you know of the Visual Angle.
9. What do you call the smallest conceivable line of light waves?
10. If a number of them were traveling side by side in the same direction what name would you give them?
11. If they were all approaching some point what name would you give them?
12. If they were leaving some point?
13. Explain Absorption.
14. What is meant by the word divergent?
15. In what direction does light leave a luminous point? That is does it go up, down, east, west, or which direction?
16. Rays leaving a luminous body do they travel parallel or not? If not, how?
17. In nature does light travel in Beams, Pencils, or in both?
18. Explain what will happen to rays of light coming in contact with a piece of plate glass.
19. Practically, rays entering the eye must come from how far in order to be divergent?

20. In order to be parallel?

21. How many times could light travel around the world in 4 seconds?

22. What effect would glass have upon its rapidity?

23. What is Transmission?

24. How many different classes of substances may light come in contact with? What are they?

25. Give an example of each not using those given in the lesson.

26. What is Refraction?

27. Which has the greatest divergence, rays from 3 inches or rays from 3 feet? Or is there any difference?

28. What is the difference between rays coming from 30 feet and those coming from 300 feet?

29. Does light travel in curves or how? Or does it have any regular mode of motion?

30. How do you know?

LESSON NO. 2

Reflection, or Catoptrics.

As WE SAW in our previous lesson, a portion of the rays falling upon a substance are thrown back into the same medium from which they came. The study of the laws which govern these rebounding rays is called "Reflecting or Catoptrics." The ray as it approaches the substance is called the "Incident Ray;" after leaving the substance it is called the "Reflected Ray." Make a heading in your notebook as follows: "REFLECTION, or CATOPTRICS," then Copy:

    17. Incident Ray is the name given to the approaching ray coming in contact with a reflecting surface.

    18. Reflected Ray is the name given to the ray rebounding from the surface.

Let us study now the movements of these Reflected Rays, so that we may be able to determine positively just what direction they will take, provided we know the direction of the Incident Rays.

If you have in your hand a ball, and throw it straight down to the ground it will return straight to your hand. If your companion is standing a short distance from you, and you wish the ball to rebound toward him, you will not throw the ball straight down but will throw it obliquely toward the ground so that it will strike just half way between yourself and him. No matter at what distance he stands you always aim to strike the ground just half way between, knowing that the ball will leave the ground at just the same angle as it struck. Likewise if you throw the ball against a building the same results will follow. If thrown perpendicular to the surface of the building it will return to you. If you hit the surface ten feet to one side your friend must stand twenty feet from you in order to receive it. It will be time well spent if during your leisure moments you take a ball and experiment with it, noticing which way it will rebound under different conditions. For instance roll it along the floor to the wall, both perpendicularly and obliquely, and watch the results. You will find that in every instance where it strikes perpendicularly it will return along the same line to your hand, and in every instance where it is thrown obliquely the angle formed by the line of direction toward the wall, and the line of direction from the wall, can be divided into two equal parts by a line drawn perpendicular to the surface of the wall, at the point where the ball touched.

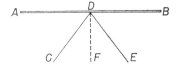

To make this more clear let us suppose that the ball in going toward the wall AB, will travel over the path CD and striking the wall at D will rebound over the path DE. Now if we draw a line DF perpendicular to the wall, from the point of contact D, the angle CDE will be cut into two equal parts, the angle CDF and FDE being of the same size.

These laws governing a rebounding body apply with equal correctness to the Reflection of Light. If you will turn to Fig. 1 in your Hartridge, you will see a diagram very similar to the one we have just been using. In this case the line AB, represents an incident ray of light, coming in contact with a plane surface CD, while BE represents the reflected ray. The perpendicular drawn to the surface at the point of contact B, cuts the angle ABE into two equal parts, making the angle ABF (which is called the Angle of Incidence) of the same size as the angle PBE (which is called the Angle of Reflection). From this we have the following rule, which although it is given in Hartridge, is of so much importance that it had better be put in the notebook also. Copy:

19. The angle of incidence is always equal to the angle of reflection.

If you do not understand every word of the foregoing explanations stop now and go over it again and again, until it is perfectly clear to you, for this Rule No. 19 is of the utmost importance in the study of every portion of this subject, and if you will learn the rule by heart and apply it to every condition that may arise in all our following considerations of Reflection, you will have mastered the secret of every phenomenon which may take place. The next rule, (also given by Hartridge) although a little difficult to explain to you on paper, is nevertheless simple. Copy:

20. The incident and reflected rays are both in the same plane which is perpendicular to the reflecting surface.

This means that the two rays, and the perpendicular line which we drew, all lie in the same plane. For instance when you rolled the ball along the floor to the wall, the floor represented the plane upon which all these lines were drawn, and you will notice that the ball in its rebound did not rise into the air and take an upward course, but simply rolled away in the same plane. Also when you threw the ball to the ground for your companion to catch, it rose again in the same plane without turning to the right or left. That is, if your friend stood directly west of you, you threw the ball west and down, and in its rebound it neither turned north nor south, but continued straight west and up, until it reached him, and a large sheet of paper standing on edge between you would have cut both the lines of descent and ascent, as well as the line drawn perpendicular to the ground. This is the point which Rule No. 20 aims to bring out and which I trust I have made clear.

The above laws apply in every instance. Light falling upon a rough uneven surface is dispersed and reflected in every direction, but only because the rough surface is made up of an infinite number of tiny planes inclined in every conceivable direction, and each ray is reflected according to the inclination of the particular plane it strikes, but is always governed by the foregoing laws. In speaking of a reflecting surface it would not be correct to simply consider a polished surface, or a mirror, but bear in mind that there is no existing substance in the universe which is not a reflecting substance, as it would be invisible to us if the light did not come from the substance to our eyes. As you look around the room then, at the different objects, try to imagine the infinite number of rays bounding and rebounding, crossing and recrossing one another, so that there is not a single moment, when every object in the room is not distinctly visible to your eye, no matter in what part of the room you may be situated.

Mirrors.

The difference between a rough uneven surface and a polished surface, lies in the fact that in the polished surface a large proportion of these tiny planes lie in the same direction, thus reflecting a great many of the rays in the same direction, and the more highly polished the surface is, the larger number of rays will be reflected alike. No surface has ever yet, or ever can be, so highly polished as not to leave some irregular planes, which will disperse a portion of the light and absorb a portion. High grade mirrors however, are as near an approach to perfection as has yet been attained. Still if you will look closely at these mirrors from an oblique position, you will see a lead-colored glow, or haze, coming from the mercurial coating on the back of the glass, and will also see the glass itself. These would not be visible were it not for the fact that some of the rays are dispersed and thus come to your eye. However the great majority of these rays undergo a uniform reflection and so few of them are dispersed or absorbed that we may practically consider a good mirror as a perfect reflecting surface.

Mirrors are divided into two classes, plane and curved.

An ordinary looking-glass is an example of a plane mirror, and rays of light coming in contact with it will be thrown off according to the laws which are covered by Rules 19 and 20. For instance if you stand with your face directly in front of a plane mirror, the light from your eye will go straight to the mirror and will be reflected straight back to your eye again, so that you will see your eye in all its detail, size, color, expression and everything just as other people see it. In this case the reflection takes place in just the same manner as when the ball was thrown straight against the building, and returned straight to your hand. Considering it according to Rule 19, we will see that as the ray went from your eye to the glass, straight along the line of perpendicular, there could be no angle formed WITH the perpendicular, as the line of direction and the perpendicular are one and the same. Hence the Angle of incidence must be equal to 0 (nothing), and by Rule 19, the angles of incidence and Reflection being equal, the angle of reflection in this case must also be equal to 0, and the reflected ray will return along the perpendicular without forming an angle of any kind. Our rule then still holds good in this case as well as in others.

Let us now consider some of the other rays which leave your eye and strike the mirror at some other point, for we learned in Lesson No. 1, that rays leaving an object travel off in every direction. For instance a certain ray leaves your eye taking a direction to the right, striking the mirror at a distance of two feet to the right of where the previous ray touched it. It must be clear to you by Rule 19, that a person standing by your side must be just four feet from you to catch that particular ray. If he stands five feet from you he will catch a ray which touched the mirror at a distance of two and one-half feet from the first ray, and so on, so that no matter where he stands he will be able to receive some ray which has started from your eye or from any other portion of your face. At the same time rays will leave his face striking the mirror at every point and you will in turn be able to receive a portion of them regardless of the position either of you may occupy. Rule 19 has however still asserted itself, never failing in its correctness. You may stand close before the mirror and your friend may go back to the extreme end of the room, yet the same law holds good. Let CD represent a plane mirror, the point A representing your eye and the point B the eye of your friend. The

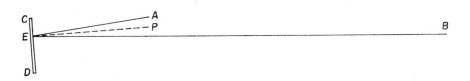

ray from your eye travels over the line AE, strikes the mirror at E, and is reflected over the line EB, continuing in a straight line until at last it is intercepted by your friend's eye. If you draw a perpendicular PE, at the point of contact E you will find that the two angles are just of a size, the same as in all the previous instances. Reversing the directions, a ray coming from your friend's eye over the path BE will continue straight until it comes in contact with the mirror when it will be reflected over the path EA, and will be received by yourself. You will both therefore, be able at all times to see one another by looking in the direction of the mirror.

Image Formed by a Plane Mirror.

Having considered the reflection of a single ray by a plane mirror, we will now consider a number of rays collectively. Instead of your friend standing in front of the mirror, let us take some object, as an arrow, and place it before the glass. Rays coming from

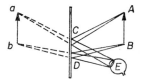

the point A, will diverge in every direction. Part of them will take the direction AG, and will be reflected to the eye over the line CE. Our eyes only being accustomed to judging of straight lines are unable to comprehend the change of direction which the rays have undergone by the reflection, and can only consider them as having come from a distance back of the mirror at "a." Rays coming from B will be reflected at D toward the eye over the line DE. Again the eye is unable to comprehend the change, and instantly assumes that the rays come from the back of the mirror at "b." The rays from A (one of the extreme points of the arrow) and those from B (the other extreme point of the arrow) form in the eye an angle CED, which according to Rule 12 is called the Visual Angle, and as we saw in Lesson No. 1, the Visual Angle is the measure by which the eye judges of size and distance, the arrow is immediately considered by the eye to be situated back of the mirror at the same distance which it is really placed in front of the mirror, the size appearing the same as the actual size of the arrow.

In this case the eye only errs regarding the direction of the object, its judgment of the size and of the distance which the light has traveled being perfectly accurate. We shall find instances as we proceed in our studies, where the eye is not only deceived regarding direction, but regarding size and distance as well. In the plane mirror however, direction alone is misleading.

In the above demonstration, the real arrow receives the name of "Object," the imaginary arrow which appears back of the mirror being called the "Image." As this "Image" is only imaginary and does not really exist, it is called an "Unreal," or "Virtual Image," Copy:

21. A Virtual Image is one which is only imaginary and does not really exist.

In these foregoing considerations, we have found that the image formed by a plane mirror is situated back of the mirror, the same distance that the object is situated in front of the mirror; that it is of the same size as the object; and that it is unreal or Virtual. We may then deduct the following rule. Copy:

22. The image formed by a plane mirror is Virtual; of the same size as the object; and is situated at a distance back of the mirror, equal to the distance of the object in front of the mirror.

By forming a habit of observation you will be surprised how many examples of reflection will come under your notice at all times and at all places. As you pass a store window, you will not only see the interior of the store, but will see a reflection of yourself in the glass, the occupants of the store at the same time seeing you also. This is an evidence of the truth of our statement made in Lesson No. 1 that a portion of the light striking a transparent substance, would be transmitted, and another portion reflected. Stand upon the bank of a pond, and upon the opposite side you will not only see the trees standing upright, but also images of the trees hanging tops down, below the surface of the water. By this you know that rays of light from the tree-tops have come down obliquely, striking the water's surface a short distance from you, and been reflected upward again toward your eye. If you will make it a point to take notice of all these phenomena, and each time think out in your own mind just what course the rays must take in order to produce the different results, you will become a master of this subject, and reflection of light with all its curious illusions, will be as simple to you as the alphabet.

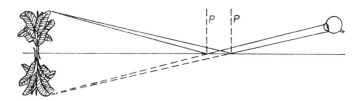

In our next lesson we will take up Curved Mirrors and will finish the study of Reflection. For your study between mails you will begin at "Reflection by a Concave Surface," Page 3 of Hartridge, and end at "Refraction" on Page 6. Also go over the first three pages again, and see if you do not find them much more simple and easy to understand than you did before.

(End of Lesson No. 2.)

QUESTIONS ON LESSON NO. 2.

31. What is an Incident Ray?
32. What name is given to the ray which is thrown off from a reflecting surface?
33. Explain the meaning of Rule 19.
34. Of Rule 20.
35. If these rules are correct, why is it that light goes in every direction from unpolished surfaces?
36. What is a reflecting surface?
37. What is a polished surface, and in what way does it differ from an unpolished one?
38. How many kinds of mirrors are there, and what are they?
39. Give an example of a plane mirror not using the one given in the lesson.
40. What happens to a ray of light which strikes the mirror exactly perpendicular to the surface of the mirror?
41. If it strikes obliquely?
42. What is an image?
43. What kind of an image is formed by a plane mirror?
44. Why?
45. Where is the image, formed by a plane mirror, situated?
46. How does the image in a plane mirror compare with the object in size, distance, direction, etc.

EXPLANATIONS ON LESSONS NO. 1 AND NO. 2.

1. In answering this question I suppose some of you said that Light is Luminiferous Aether; others that it is a wave motion and perhaps others that it is an agent of vision. Neither of these would be good answers. Light is not luminiferous aether nor a wave motion and if you should tell your friend that it is an agent of vision, I am afraid he would know but very little more about it than he did before. The best definition that I know of is as follows: Light is a sensation produced upon the retina of the eye by waves of luminiferous aether striking against it. Notice the first four words of this definition: "Light is a Sensation." In other words it is simply a feeling, just as pain or taste is a feeling. We throw a stone across the street at a dog. The stone flying through the air is not called "pain," but when it strikes the dog, the FEELING or SENSATION that it produces upon the dog is carried along the nerves to the brain and the FEELING is called pain. We can also say that a wave of luminiferous aether traveling through space is not light for luminiferous aether is an invisible vapor, but if it enters the eye and strikes the inner lining or retina, the FEELING that it produces is carried along the optic nerve to the brain and we call it "Light." We can produce the same feeling by closing the lids and rubbing the eye-ball or we produce it when we fall and strike our head on the ice or pavement. We call it "seeing stars," but we are really only jarring the retina and producing upon it the feeling called Light.

2. Luminiferous aether is all about us at all times. If we are in a closed, dark room, the room is full of aether, but it is motionless. If we apply a match to the gas jet we have a flame, every particle of which is in rapid vibration caused by the chemical action of combustion. This constant motion of all the little particles of which the flame is composed must quickly set the aether into motion, just as beating your hand rapidly in the water would

set the water into motion. The waves of aether are now keeping up a constant beating against the retina and we say the room is illuminated. Turn off the gas and the movement ceases, the aether once more stands motionless and we say the room is dark. The same is true of any other luminous body, as the Sun, a lamp, an electric light, a firefly, etc. All of these substances set the aether into motion because every particle of which they are composed is itself in motion.

3. Any substance or body that is capable of disturbing the aether sufficient to cause waves, is called a Luminous Body.

4. Other bodies from which we get light are "NOT LUMINOUS," or, to use a latin term, "NON LUMINOUS" bodies.

5. Non-luminous bodies do not cause a wave motion of the aether themselves, but simply reflect the wave back again when it strikes against them. The answer to this question then should be: By Reflection.

6. I expect that every one of the class answered this question something like this: "The Moon, a mirror, a piece of polished metal, etc." While all of these are good examples it is not necessary to confine them to polished surfaces, nor heavenly bodies. A cow, or a pig, or a stick of wood, or a book would be equally good. Really any body that is not luminous is, of course, a non luminous body, and any object that we can see must be a reflecting body for we would not be able to see it at all if light waves were not reflected from it to our eyes.

7. Reflecting is the "rebounding" of light waves. Just as a ball rebounds when thrown against a hard substance.

8. The Visual Angle is an angle (or corner) formed by rays of light from the extreme points of an object entering and meeting in the eye. This angle is narrowed or widened as the object is smaller or larger, or, as it is carried farther away or closer to the eye. The use of this angle is to enable the eye to judge of size, or distance.

9. According to Rule No. 1 it is called a Ray.   10. According to Rule No. 3 it is called a Beam.   11. A converging pencil.

12. A diverging pencil.

13. Absorption is the destruction of light waves, caused either by contact with a substance, or passing through a substance.

14. Two or more rays starting from a point and gradually separating from one another.

15. Light goes in EVERY direction from any luminous point.

16. If they travel in EVERY direction they cannot be parallel for the word parallel means side by side in the SAME direction. Hence, the answer should be: "Diverging."

17. As they travel diverging they must travel in pencils, although if they come to us from infinity, we call them parallel, or beams. Strictly speaking however, they are still pencils.

18. Part will be absorbed, part reflected and part transmitted.

19. They are practically divergent only when they come to us from a distance of less than six meters.

20. Six meters or more.

21. Strictly speaking it could not travel around the world at all, because light does not travel in circles and because it could not travel so far through air without being absorbed. It could travel in open space a distance equal to about 29 times around the world in that length of time.

22. It would be retarded while passing through the glass, but the instant it emerges on the opposite side it resumes its old rate of speed.

23. In Optics, the act of passing through.   24. Three: Transparent, Translucent and Opaque.   25. Respectively, Alcohol, China, Brick.

26. The bending of a ray of light in going from one substance into another of different density.   27. Those coming from 3 inches (Rule 4).   28. Practically no difference (Rule 6).

29. Always in straight lines while in the same medium.

30. Because we cannot see around a corner. Or, because we can see objects through a long straight tube but if the tube be bent the rays cannot follow the bend of the tube and come to our eyes.

31. The name given to the original ray.   32. It is called a Reflected Ray.   33. It means that if a ray strikes a surface at an angle of 40 degrees with the perpendicular it will be reflected at an angle of 40 degrees on the other side of perpendicular.

34. It means that the reflected ray will be exactly on the opposite side of the perpendicular from the incident ray.

35. Because an unpolished surface is made up of a great many independent surfaces, each one acting according to the inclination at which it stands. 36. Any surface that we can see.

37. A polished surface is an unbroken surface. It differs from an unpolished one as a rifle differs from a shot gun. It throws all of the light in a solid bunch, while the unpolished surface scatters it.

38. Two general classes. Plane and Curved.   39. Any polished metal that is perfectly flat. A pond of water.   40. It returns over to the same path that it came.   41. It forms an angle of reflection equal to the angle of incidence.   42. A duplicate, or likeness of an object.

43. Unreal or "Virtual."   44. Because it is only imagination.

45. Behind the mirror equal to the distance of the object in front of it.   46. The same except DIRECTION. The object in front of the glass while the image is behind it.

L E S S O N N O. 3.

Reflection, by Curved Mirrors.

CURVED MIRRORS may be Spherical, Cylindrical, or of other forms. The ones with which we shall have most to do, however, are the spherical, both concave and convex.

An ordinary glass lamp reflector is a good example of a spherical mirror. If you have one handy take it and examine the surfaces. The inner or hollow surface is a concave spherical mirror, while the opposite surface, or back, is a convex spherical mirror. Let us study what effect these surfaces may have upon rays of light which may chance to come in contact with them.

In any instance of reflection we know that if we are told the direction of the incident ray, and can draw a perpendicular to the point of contact, it will be a very easy matter by Rule 19 to draw the reflected ray, having only to draw it in such a manner that the Angle of reflection on that side of the perpendicular will be equal to the angle of incidence on the other side. "But," you say, "how can a line be drawn perpendicular to a surface which has a continuous curve, no two points having the same inclination?" Our only solution of this problem is to draw a separate perpendicular for each and every point with which rays come in contact. Let us see how this may be done. If you wish to draw a circle, or a portion of a circle, upon the blackboard you will use a piece of chalk and a string. Placing the end of the string at a certain point and holding it firmly, you will with the chalk tied at the other end describe a circle, or curve, by holding the string tight and sweeping the chalk across the board. Your curve will then appear as shown in Fig. 1, with the point C, where you held the string, representing

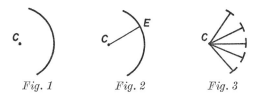

| *Fig. 1* | *Fig. 2* | *Fig. 3* |

the center of the circle, or curve. Now if you will draw a line or radius, from the center to any point on the curve (as C E Fig. 2) the line drawn will be the perpendicular to that particular point of the curve where it comes in contact with it. That is, the line CE in Fig. 2, is perpendicular to the point E of the curve. In other words let us imagine that a curved surface is made up of an infinite number of tiny planes, regularly inclined as shown in Fig. 3. As you will readily see, a line drawn from the center of curvature C, to any of these planes is always perpendicular to that plane. From this we can deduct the following rule which will enable us to follow the reflected rays as readily in dealing with curved surfaces as when considering plane surfaces. Copy:

23. *The perpendicular to any point of a curved spherical mirror is a line drawn from that point to the center of curvature of the mirror.*

Let us now study the effects produced by a concave mirror upon rays coming from different distances.

We saw in Lesson No. 1 that the rays coming from a distance of twenty feet or more were considered parallel. In Fig. 4 the curve A B represents a concave mirror with C as its center of curvature and the lines D E, G H, and J K, three parallel rays of

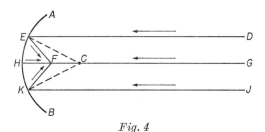

Fig. 4

light. To find in what direction the ray D E will be reflected we have simply to draw a perpendicular C E from the center to the point E, and so draw the reflected ray that the angles of incidence and reflection will be of the same size. This throws the reflected ray in the direction E F. By the same reasoning the ray J K will be reflected in the direction K F. The ray G H having struck the mirror exactly perpendicular to the point of contact will be reflected straight back over the line H F. You will notice that all these rays were reflected toward the point F, and that all met at that point. This would be as true of a large number of rays as of three. This point F where the rays meet is called a focus. Copy:

24. *A focus is a point where two or more rays of light meet.*

In the above case the rays under consideration were parallel rays. In order that we may distinguish between the focus for parallel rays and any other focus which may come up in our studies, this focus for parallel rays has been given the name of "Principal Focus" so that hereafter when we speak of the principal focus you may know at once that the focus for parallel rays is the one referred to. Make a heading in your notebook like this: "CONCAVE MIRRORS." Then copy:

25. *The principal focus of a concave mirror is that point where rays which were parallel before reflection, will meet each other after reflection.*

26. *The distance of the principal focus from the mirror is called the focal length of the mirror.*

27. *The principal focus of a concave mirror is situated half way between the mirror and its center of curvature.*

Having considered the reflection of rays coming from infinity (6 meters or more), let us bring the object up to a Finite Distance (less than 6 meters) and follow the reflected rays. As we learned in Lesson No. 1, these rays will be diverging. Let A B, Fig. 5, represent a concave mirror with C as its center and F its principal focus. If we place our object at 0, rays will proceed from it over the lines O E, O D, and O H. Drawing our perpendicular from the center C, to each point of contact E, D and H, we can

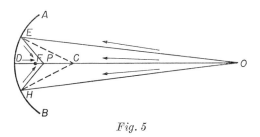

Fig. 5

draw the reflected rays as before, according to Rule 19, and we find them coming to a focus at P between the principal focus and the center. Notice now what has happened.

In the first place the object was placed at infinity, and the rays met at the principal focus, half way between the center and the mirror; next, the object was brought nearer to the mirror and its focus moved from the principal focus toward the center. The object and the focus then are approaching one another and if this is continued must eventually meet. The question is, at what point will this meeting take place? If we move the object still nearer as in Fig. 6, the focus has again moved toward the center but not so rapidly as the object. Let us next move our object exactly to the center and see what will take place. We know that a line drawn from the center to any portion of the mirror is always perpendicular to the point of contact. Rays then, leaving the center must strike the mirror perpendicularly at every point, and will of course be reflected straight back over the same lines to the center again, coming to a focus there. (See Fig. 7.) Object and focus have met then exactly at the center of curvature.

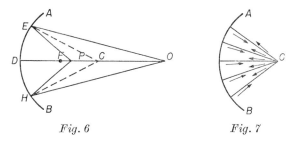

Fig. 6   Fig. 7

If we still continue to move the object closer to the mirror, where will the focus be situated? Turning again to Fig. 6, let us suppose the object to be placed at P instead of O. By drawing our perpendiculars from C as before, and following Rule 19 we find that the reflected rays will be thrown off in the direction of O, just the reverse of what happened when the object was at O. It would appear then that these two points O and P bear a reciprocal relation to one another, so that if we place the object at O the focus will be at P, or if we place the object at P the image, or focus, will be at O. This relationship of the two points to one another has been named "Conjugate," so that we may say that O is a conjugate of P, or that P is a conjugate of O. Copy:

    28. Any two points so situated that if an object be placed at one of them, its focus, or image, will be at the other, are called "Conjugate Foci."

(The word "foci," pronounced "fo-si," is the plural for focus. Thus we would say "two foci," not "two focusses.")

If we still continue to move the object closer to the mirror the focus will continue to move away. Hence if we place the object at P, Fig. 5, the image (or conjugate focus) will travel off to O, moving faster now than the object, until at last we reach the principal focus, when by Fig. 4 if the rays leave F, they will strike the mirror and be reflected off along the lines ED, HG and KJ, parallel to each other, toward infinity.

In the following these movements you will have noticed that light in leaving one point and approaching another, always travels over the same paths that it would take were the points reversed and the light traveling from the second point to the first. This law of reciprocity is true in all the studies of optics no matter with what subject we are dealing. Copy:

29. *In all considerations of optics, light leaving one point and approaching another, will always travel over the same paths that it would follow in leaving the second point and approaching the first.*

To review this subject we have learned, first, that light coming from infinity will be reflected by the concave mirror to a point half way from the mirror to the center, called the principal focus; second, that light coming from a finite distance, beyond the center will come to a point between the principal focus and the center, called its conjugate focus; third, that light coming from the center of curvature to the mirror will be reflected straight back over the same lines to the center again; fourth, that light coming from a point between the center and the principal focus, will have its conjugate focus between the center and infinity; and fifth, that light coming from the principal focus will be reflected back in parallel rays. There is now but one other condition to consider. Viz.: When the object is brought still closer to the mirror than the principal focus, in other words when it is brought between the principal focus and the mirror. Heretofore as we have brought the object toward the mirror, the focus has been traveling from the mirror, until as we reached the principal focus, the focus had reached infinity. Now as we bring the object still closer to the mirror what will happen? Perhaps you will say that the focus has moved away to beyond infinity. But can that be possible? Infinity means twenty feet or more, and that word "more" implies as far beyond 20 feet as you can imagine, so that no matter how great the distance it will still remain "infinity." How, then can we dispose of the focus? Let AB Fig. 8 represent

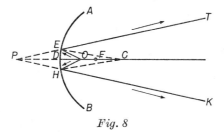

Fig. 8

a concave mirror, C the center, and F the principal focus. If we place the object at O, between the mirror and the principal focus, the ray striking the mirror at E will be reflected according to Rule 19 toward T, and the ray OH toward K. The rays then will leave the mirror diverging (though not so diverging as before reflection) and can never come to a focus. We can however by tracing the reflected rays backward over the dotted lines EP and HP, come to a point where the rays appear to have started from. This point we call the unreal or "Negative" focus. Hence when the object is brought closer than the principal focus, its focus is a "Negative" focus situated back of the mirror.

These points are a little complicated but if you will go over them carefully, step by step, several times before going any farther, it will soon become clear.

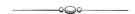

Thus far we have only considered concave mirrors in their principal or primary axis. That is, the object was always at some point directly facing the mirror. For instance: in Fig. 4 the line GH was the principal axis of the mirror; in Figs. 5, 6 and 8, OD was the principal axis, and you will notice that in each instance the focus was always situated somewhere on that axis. In Fig. 9, the object is not situated upon the principal axis but is placed at one side at O. In this case the OD drawn from the object to the mirror

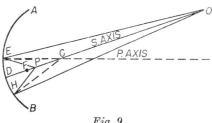

Fig. 9

through the center C, forms an axis, which in order to distinguish it from the principal axis, has been given the name of "Secondary axis," and the object placed upon a point of this axis will have its focus at some point on the same axis according to the same laws which we have just considered. We can then, deduct the following rule. Copy:

    30. The focus formed by a concave mirror is always found on the same axis as the object, whether principal or secondary.

Images Formed by Concaved Mirrors.

Having learned to find the focus for a single point, we have only to consider a number of points collectively in order to create an image. Let the arrow XZ Fig. 10 represent an object, and AB a concave mirror with C as its center. The point X of the arrow is

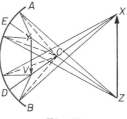

Fig. 10

situated on the secondary axis XD, and will have its focus on that axis at V. The point Z is situated on the secondary axis ZE and will have its focus on that axis at Y. In the same manner all points of the arrow between X and Z will have their foci in regular order between V and Y, so that we have a perfect inverted image of the arrow XZ at VY, smaller than the object.

If the arrow is at infinity the image will be the principal focus; if at a finite distance, the image is at its conjugate. If we place the arrow at the center the image will also be at the center, inverted and the same size as the object. If we place the object nearer than the center (for instance let us call VY Fig. 10 the object), the image will be inverted, larger than the object, and beyond the center (as at XZ). So far none of these images are imaginary, (or virtual) but do really exist, as the light is actually thrown to focus at these points, and if you will hold a card in correct position it will receive the light and show you a perfect inverted picture of the object. These images therefore are called "Real Images."

If we continue to move the arrow closer until we reach the principal focus the rays, as we have learned, will leave the mirror parallel and there will be no image, for, parallel rays can never come to a focus but will alway continue parallel. Moving the arrow still nearer the mirror we have, Fig. 11, DG representing the object and AB the mirror. Rays from D will be reflected diverging, (see Fig. 8) toward the eye E, as will also rays

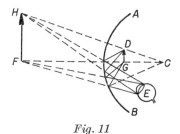

Fig. 11

from G. Carrying D's rays backward to the point from which they appear to come, we have a negative focus of D back of the mirror at H. Likewise we have a negative focus of G at F. Hence we will have an Enlarged; Upright; Virtual image of the arrow DG at HF, which will decrease in size as the object continues to approach the mirror. Instead of having therefore, as in the case of plane mirrors, only one condition, viz.: the image always virtual, of the same size as the object, and upright, we have in concave mirrors a number of different results, each depending entirely upon the position of the object. At times the image is real, inverted and smaller than the object, at others it is real, inverted and larger than the object; again it may be inverted, real, and of the same size as the object, or upright, virtual and larger than the object; and under yet another condition, there will be no image at all. Our mirror then which at first thought would seem so simple, has proved itself to be a very complicated instrument furnishing material for unlimited study and investigation. The following rules will cover the different changes which take place. Copy:

31. *In a concave mirror, if the object is placed infinity, the image will be real, inverted, smaller than the object, and at the principal focus of the mirror.*

32. *If the object is at some finite distance beyond the center of curvature, the image will be real, inverted, smaller than the object, and between the principal focus and the center.*

33. *If the object is at the center of curvature the image will be real, inverted, same size as the object and at the same place.*

34. *If the object is between the center of curvature and the principal focus, the image will be real, inverted, larger than the object, and beyond the center.*

35. *If the object is at the principal focus there will be no image.*

36. *If the object is between the principal focus and the mirror, the image is virtual, enlarged, upright, and back of the mirror. As the object continues to approach the mirror the image decreases until the object reaches the mirror, when the image is of the same size.*

Take your lamp reflector now and prove these rules. Bring it very close to your face and the reflection will be upright and considerably magnified; draw it slowly away and the face in the glass will gradually increase in size, until you reach the principal focus, when the image entirely disappears. Continue to draw the mirror away and you will see your face inverted, constantly decreasing in size as the mirror moves away. Many useful articles are based upon these principles. For instance, the lamp reflector is placed so that the blaze is just at the principal focus of the mirror. What happens? Rays from the flame will strike the mirror and be reflected parallel, thus causing a beam of light to be thrown off in any direction you may choose to turn the mirror.

Spherical Convex Mirrors.

In convex mirrors a ray from infinity, as AB Fig. 12 will strike the mirror at B. Drawing our perpendicular from the center C, we find the ray will be reflected in the direction J. In the same manner IG will be reflected toward K. DE striking the mirror perpendicular will be thrown straight back and we therefore find that rays which come to the mirror parallel will leave the mirror diverging. Carrying these diverging rays backward, to

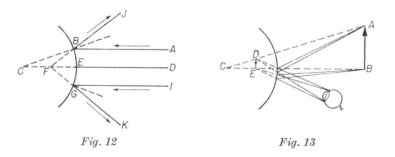

Fig. 12   Fig. 13

the point from which they appear to have come, we find a negative principal focus at F half way between the mirror and the center. Rays coming from a finite distance being diverging, the reflected rays will of course be more diverging than before, and the negative conjugate focus will be between the negative principal focus and the mirror, and the closer the object is brought the nearer will the focus be to the surface of the mirror.

What is true of one point will be equally true of many points. If we place an arrow in front of a convex mirror as AB Fig. 13, we will find the negative focus for the point A situated at D, and that for B situated at E. We have then an upright, virtual image of AB at DE, smaller than the object, and situated back of the mirror between the principal focus and the mirror. The following rules will cover the conditions arising in the convex mirror. Copy: *"CONVEX MIRRORS."*

37. *The image of a convex mirror is always virtual, upright, and situated back of the mirror but never farther back than the principal focus.*

38. *The image is always smaller than the object except when the object touches the mirror, at which time object and image are of the same size.*

These rules you can prove by looking in the back of your lamp reflector.

Cylindrical Mirrors.

The name of these mirrors indicates their shape. They are simply convex or concave in one direction, while at right angles to that direction they are straight, or plane. Your lead pencil is perfectly straight the long way, but considered in a cross direction it is round, or curved. The same is true of cylindrical mirrors. You have seen them no doubt many times. They give one's image the appearance of being very short and very wide, or else very tall and very lean. These distortions are easily explained. The direction of the mirror which is straight is a plane mirror and you are reflected in that direction, perfectly natural. The opposite direction being curved, will enlarge or diminish your image, as the case may be, in that direction, making the image, for instance, very short in the vertical direction, while laterally the size is exact.

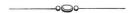

This lesson, which I consider the most complicated and difficult of the whole series concludes the study of Reflection. Go over it carefully and thoroughly, taking plenty of time, and by all means learn it well. If you do, you will have gotten a firm hold of the elementary principles of the optical science, and your success in the work will always be greater for your earnest study at this time.

For your study between mails review the entire subject of Reflection as given by Hartridge, also beginning at "Refraction" on Page 6, study to "Refraction by Lenses," Page 11.

(*End of Lesson No. 3.*)

QUESTIONS ON LESSON NO. 3.

47. How do you draw a perpendicular to some point on a concave mirror?

48. How far from the mirror will the center of curvature be, if the focal length of the mirror is 9 inches?

49. Give your understanding of conjugate foci.

50. If with a concave mirror having its center 14 inches from its surface, we place an object 7 inches from its surface where will the image be?

51. If with a concave mirror whose focal length is 6 inches we place an object a foot from the mirror, where will the image be?

52. If with the same mirror the object be placed **3** inches from the surface, tell me about the image.

53. If placed 8 inches from the mirror?

54. Rule **33** says that if the object is placed at the center, the image will be inverted. Is this correct? I would think that if rays from every point of the object were thrown back point for point, the image would be upright, the same as the object. Is there a flaw in the rule, or what is the trouble?

55. How many kinds of images can be produced by a concave mirror and what are they?

56. In concave mirrors, where must the object be in order to have the image larger than the object, and inverted?

57. In order to have the image larger than the object, and upright?

58. Is there any point at which the object may be placed, to produce a real image of the same size as the object?

59. At what point will you place the object to produce a virtual image of the same size as the object?

60. Tell what you know concerning the images produced by convex mirrors.

61. Tell me the shape, position, etc., of a mirror which will make your image appear very short, very wide, and upside down.

LESSON NO. 4.

Refraction, or Dioptrics.

IF A BEAM of light comes in contact with a transparent substance, a portion of the rays will be absorbed, another portion reflected, and still another portion transmitted. If the beam strikes the substance perpendicular to its surface the transmitted rays will pass straight into it without any change of direction. If, however, the beam strikes the transparent substance obliquely the transmitted rays will, at the moment of entering, be deviated, or bent out of their regular path and will travel in the new medium at a greater or less angle from the direction they had previously taken. Let M, Fig. 1 represent a vessel of water, and AB a ray of light striking the water's surface obliquely at B. The ray instead of continuing straight toward D is bent, or refracted at the point of entrance and takes the direction BC. On the other hand, if the beam were traveling in the opposite direction (that is from the water to the air over the path CB) it would be bent (or refracted) in the direction BA instead of continuing in the direction BE. We can therefore say, that light passing obliquely from one medium into another, will be bent, or refracted, out of its original course. If you will take an empty cup and place in it a coin in such a position that it will be just hidden from your view by the cup's

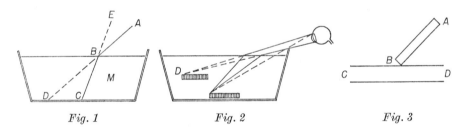

| Fig. 1 | Fig. 2 | Fig. 3 |

rim and slowly fill the cup with water without disturbing the coin, you will find that the coin will gradually appear in view, until it will be wholly visible. A glance at Fig. 2 will explain this phenomenon. The unbroken lines represent the rays as they actually travel from the coin to the eye, being so bent at the surface of the water that they appear to the eye as having come from the point D.

The study of the laws governing this bending or refracting of the rays of light is called "Refraction, or Dioptrics." In order that we may understand how a ray of light is bent by passing from one medium to another, let us imagine AB Fig. 3 to be a ray of light (greatly magnified) approaching the surface CD. It is evident that the lower or right hand side of this ray will strike the surface before the upper or left side can do so. We learned in Lesson No. 1, that light traveling in a dense medium, would proceed more slowly than when traveling in a rare medium; that is, the rapidity will be lessened. The lower right hand corner therefore entering the water first will be retarded in its progress, while the opposite corner, still remaining in air, will continue at its former rate of speed until it, too reaches the surface of the water, when the entire ray will be submerged, and will travel again in a straight line, but at a less rapid rate than when it was traveling through the air. You can readily understand that the left side of the ray, gaining as it does, upon the right at the time of entering the water, will bend the ray so that it will proceed in a steeper direction than before, as shown in Fig. 1. On the other hand, if the ray was leaving the water in the direction CB, Fig. 1, the upper left corner of the ray entering the air first would gain upon the opposite side, which is still

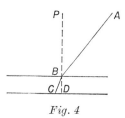

Fig. 4

in the water, and the result would be that the ray would be bent in the direction BA.

If we will draw a perpendicular PB to the surface of the water at the point of contact B, Fig. 4, we will notice that the ray in entering the water is bent (or refracted) closer to the perpendicular than before, or if we consider it as coming from the water into the air, it will be bent farther from the perpendicular than when it was in the water. We can therefore deduct the following rules, which will apply in every instance of refraction which may come before us in our studies. Copy:

    39. When light passes perpendicularly from one medium to another, it is not refracted.

    40. When light passes obliquely from a rarer to a denser medium, it is refracted toward the perpendicular.

    41. When light passes obliquely from a denser to a rarer medium, it is refracted from the perpendicular.

The amount of deviation which the ray undergoes, depends, of course, upon the density of the two mediums. If the denser medium is one which will lessen the rapidity of light considerably, it will of course, refract the rays much more than if its density were only slight. In order therefore to determine just how much a ray will be bent in passing from one medium into another, it is necessary that we have a method of knowing the relative density of the two mediums. By taking the refractive power of air as the unit of refraction and calling it 1, it has been found that the refracting power of water is one and one-third times as great as that of air; the refracting power of glass one and one-half times as great as that of air; and so on. In order to express the different powers of each, we say: "The index of refraction of air is 1; the index of refraction of water is 1.3 (one and one-third); that of glass 1.5 (one and one-half), etc." Copy:

    42. The index of refraction of any substance, is its refractive power as compared with air, expressed numerically.

To make this more clear, let us consider Fig. 5. The upper part of the circle marked A represent the medium air, and the lower part of W represents water. The ray BC forms with the perpendicular PD, an angle which measures from the point B to the perpendicular, 4 equal parts. The ray striking the water at C is refracted toward the perpendicular, forming an angle which measures from the point E to the perpendicular, 3 equal parts. The angle of incidence BCP is therefore one and one-third times as large as the angle of refraction ECD. Hence we say that the index of refraction of water is 1.3. The more

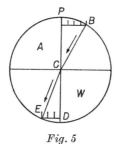

Fig. 5

obliquely the ray strikes upon the surface of the other medium the greater will be its refraction, for we can readily see that if the angle of refraction always maintains an exact proportion to the size of the angle of incidence, that the greater the angle of incidence the greater will be the angle of refraction. It is important that we remember this for our understanding of refraction by lenses depends in a great measure upon the knowledge of this fact. Copy:

43. The greater the obliquity of the incident ray, the greater will be its refraction.

————————o◯o————————

Having studied the refraction of light in passing from one medium to another of different density, thus undergoing one change, let us now consider light passing entirely through a dense medium and emerging upon the other side. This will necessarily involve two changes instead of one, the ray passing into the denser substance constituting one change, and its emergence upon the other side constituting the other. We will first consider a substance whose two surfaces are parallel to one another. A piece of plate glass is a good example. In Fig. 6 Page 6 of your Hartridge, we know that the ray HK striking the glass at its upper surface exactly perpendicular to that surface will, by Rule 39, pass straight into the glass without being refracted in the least. As the lower surface of the glass is parallel to the upper surface, a line that is perpendicular to one must also be perpendicular to the other. Hence the ray HK will emerge into the air perpendicular to the lower surface and will not of course be refracted. The ray has therefore passed completely through the glass without undergoing any change in its direction. The ray AB however, in the same diagram strikes the surface obliquely and is refracted toward the perpendicular (Rule 40) taking the direction BC in passing through the glass. As it emerges upon the other side, it is bent or refracted FROM the perpendicular (Rule 41) and as the relation of glass to air is just the same at both surfaces, it will be refracted at exactly the same angle that it was at the time of entrance. You will therefore see that the ray after emerging from the glass will take a direction CD precisely parallel to its original direction, the only change being a lateral displacement. That is it will be slightly to one side, but traveling in the same direction that it would have taken had it not been intercepted by the glass. A glance at the dotted line at the right of the ray CD will make this clear. You will also see by the ray BE of the same diagram that a portion of the rays, instead of entering the glass, were reflected, according to Rule 19. Still another portion are absorbed, thus proving the statement made in Lesson No. 1 that rays striking a transparent substance are partially reflected, partially absorbed and partially transmitted.

If the two surfaces of the denser medium are not parallel to one another the re-fraction of the rays will be different. Let our substance consist of a piece of glass thicker at one edge than at the other, as shown in Fig. 6, and we will have a good example of this condition. A glass of such form is called a "Prism."

If an incident ray AB comes in contact with the surface of the glass at B it will be refracted according to Rule 40 toward the perpendicular PE, and will pass through the glass over the path BC. At this point we must draw a perpendicular FC to the

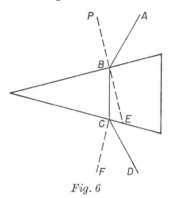

Fig. 6

lower surface of the glass. According to Rule 41, the ray as it emerges into air will be refracted from the perpendicular and will therefore take the direction CD. You will notice that at each change the ray has been bent toward the thick edge, or base, of the prism. Copy:

44. Rays passing through a prism are always refracted toward the base.

Thus far we have considered the denser mediums to be bounded by plane surfaces which, although the rays are refracted by them, do not change the relative direction which one ray bears to another. That is, if a number of rays are traveling side by side, thus forming a beam, and come in contact with one of these denser substances, each ray will be refracted exactly alike, so that when they leave the substance, although they have taken a new direction, they will still remain parallel to one another. An illustration of this is shown in Hartridge Fig. 7. Likewise, if the rays are traveling in pencils the whole pencil will be refracted alike, thus changing the general direction but not in any way disturbing the relative direction of the rays. If our denser medium is bounded by a curved surface however, the results will be different. Beams may be changed to pencils; pencils changed to more or less diverging pencils, or to beams; diverging pencils changed to converging pencils; converging to diverging; and so on. In fact the relative direction of the rays will be entirely changed, these conditions we will now consider.

Refraction by Curved Surfaces.

Let us suppose the curve AB Fig. 7, to be the bounding surface of a dense substance, the medium to the right of the curve representing glass, or water, and that to the left representing air. If a ray of light DH from an infinite distance comes in contact with the surface perpendicular to it, the ray will pass in without undergoing any refraction. Another ray EG, parallel to the first ray, coming in contact with the surface at C, will

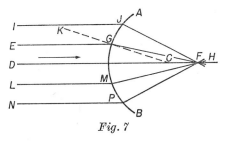

Fig. 7

not be perpendicular to it and will therefore be reflected. To ascertain in which direction it will be reflected, we must first draw a perpendicular to that point. We learned in Lesson No. 3 that the perpendicular to any point of a curved surface was a line drawn from that point to the center of curvature. We will therefore draw the perpendicular line CK. According to Rule 40, the ray will be refracted toward the perpendicular, hence will take the direction GF. The ray IJ, also parallel to the others, strikes the surface more obliquely than did the ray EG. It will therefore undergo a stronger refraction, (Rule 43), and will take the direction JF. By the same reasoning the rays LM and NP will be refracted in the direction MF and PF. Our rays then which were parallel before refraction have been changed into a converging pencil coming to a focus at the point F, and this point being the focus for rays which were parallel, we will call the principal focus.

If the rays proceed from a finite distance they will of course be diverging, and in striking the curved surface will be refracted, not to the point F, but to a point behind the principal focus. This is shown by the dotted lines diverging from G and converging to H in Hartridge Fig. 9. These two points G and H are therefore conjugate to one another and we call them "Conjugate Foci." You will see that as the luminous point is brought from infinity nearer and nearer to the curved surface, the focus is gradually moving farther and farther back until at length our luminous point reaches a place from which its rays are so diverging that the curved surface is no longer able to bring them to a focus and they travel off parallel as shown in Fig. 8. On the other hand if the rays are coming in the opposite direction, that is, if they are traveling parallel

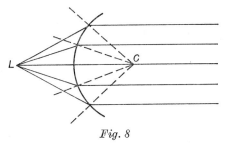

Fig. 8

from P toward the surface, they will upon emerging into the rarer medium be refracted from the perpendicular and will come to a focus at L. We have therefore two principal foci, one in front of the surface (L Fig. 8) the other behind the surface (F Fig. 7). To the one in front we give name "Anterior Principal Focus"; the other we call the "Posterior Principal Focus." These two words, Anterior and Posterior, will be used very frequently in our studies and it is necessary that the meaning of them be understood. Anterior simply means front, while posterior means back, or rear. If the luminous point be brought still nearer, between the anterior principal focus and the surface, as shown in Hartridge Fig. 10, the rays will be so diverging that the curved surface has not sufficient refractive power to even bend them parallel and they will enter the new medium still diverging, though not so much so as before. As these rays are neither directed toward a point at a finite distance, nor even toward infinity, as in the case of parallel rays, we say that they are directed toward a point "beyond infinity." Although this expression is in itself an absurdity, we find the use of it a very convenient means of expressing the destination of diverging rays, and have therefore adopted it simply as a convenience. Thus we say that diverging rays start from a finite distance and travel toward a point beyond infinity; converging rays start from a point beyond infinity and approach a point at a finite distance; parallel rays start from a point at infinity and travel toward a point at infinity; and so on.

Our rays then in Hartridge Fig. 10 enter the second medium diverging, and (to use the expression) would come to a focus beyond infinity. As such a point is not within our reach, or comprehension, we have to be content with tracing the rays backward to the point from which they appear to have come. Although this method of finding a focus is a negative one, it enables us to ascertain just the amount of divergence of the rays, and we therefore say that the focus of the point O is a negative focus situated at L. We find then in our consideration of refraction by curved surfaces, that conditions exist very similar to those found in the study of concave mirrors. For instance if the luminous point be placed at infinity its focus will be at the (posterior) principal focus; if placed at a point nearer than infinity its conjugate focus will move farther from the surface; if placed at the (anterior) principal focus the rays will leave the surface parallel; and if placed between the principal focus and the surface there will be a negative focus. The only difference between the action of the concave mirror, and that of the convex refracting surface, is this: In the mirror all rays are thrown back toward the direction from which they came, while in refraction they pass through and continue in the same general direction. As a result of this difference we will find that the focus will always be situated in the one case upon just the opposite side from where it would be in the other. For instance, in the concave mirror all the real foci are situated in front of the mirror, while in the case of refraction they will be situated back of the surface; with the concave mirror all negative foci are situated back of the mirror, while in our case of refraction they are upon the same side as the object.

If the curved surface bounding the dense medium is a concave one, the effect will be different. In Fig. 9 parallel rays entering such a surface will be refracted toward the perpendicular, but as the perpendiculars are now standing in the opposite direction to what they were in the previous instance, the rays instead of being changed to a converging pencil will take the form of a diverging pencil and will of course never meet. We can only trace them back to the point F from which they appear to come. This point is called the "Negative Principal Focus." If the luminous point is brought nearer

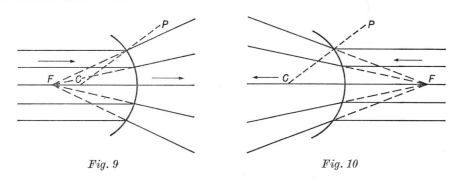

Fig. 9   Fig. 10

than infinity the rays will strike the surface diverging, and will of course be refracted more diverging than before, so that no matter at what point we place our object the focus will always be a negative one, situated in front of the surface. If the luminous point is placed on the opposite side of the surface, in the denser medium, the results will be the same. If placed at infinity, as in Fig. 10, the rays in passing from the denser to the rarer medium will be refracted from the perpendicular and will therefore diverge, having a negative principal focus at L. If placed at a finite distance, the diverging rays will be more diverging and will also have only negative foci. You will notice that with either the convex or the concave bounding surface, the rays would have precisely the same action in passing from the dense into the rare medium as when passing from the rare to the dense.

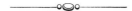

Lesson No. 5 which is devoted to the study of lenses, will end our series of lessons on physical optics. The next series will take up the anatomy and physiology of the eye and will, I trust, be less dry and more interesting than the present series. For your study between lessons, begin at "Refraction by Lenses" Page 11 and study the remainder of Chapter 1.

QUESTIONS ON LESSON NO. 4.

62. Under what conditions can a ray of light pass through a transparent substance without being refracted?
63. In what direction will light be bent in passing from air into glass?
64. In passing from water into air?
65. What is meant by "Index of Refraction"?
66. If you wish to increase the refraction of rays passing from water into air, what must be done?
67. If passing from air into water?
68. If a beam of light passes obliquely through a plate glass, what direction will it take after emerging upon the opposite side?
69. If it passes through a prism?
70. After passing through the prism will it be a beam or a pencil?
71. If rays from infinity enter a denser substance having a convex spherical surface, where will they meet?

72. Where will rays from infinity meet after leaving such a substance.

73. Tell me what you know of the conjugate foci formed by such a substance.

74. If a luminous point is placed at the posterior principal focus, what will become of the emergent rays?

75. If the substance has a concave spherical surface, tell me all you know regarding the foci.

EXPLANATIONS ON LESSONS NO. 3 AND NO. 4.

47. Every spoke in a wheel is perpendicular to the rim. Therefore a straight line drawn from any point of a curve to the center of that curve is perpendicular to that particular point. Answer: By drawing a straight line from the given point to the center of curvature of the mirror.

48. Eighteen inches. (*Rule 27.*)

49. The relationship which exists between an object and its focus. One point is always the focus of the other. (*Rule 28.*)

50. As the object is just half way between the center of curvature and the glass, it must be on the principal focus (*Rule 27*). If the object is on the principal focus, which is really the focus for parallel rays, then according to *Rule 29* the rays will be reflected parallel and never meet. Answer: there will be no image (*Rule 35*).

51. The object must be on the center of curvature (*Rule 27*). Therefore, as all rays from the center are perpendicular to the mirror as explained in Question 47, they will be reflected straight back to the center again. Answer: The image will be at the same place, of the same size, real and inverted.

52. As the principal focus is six inches away the object must now be between the principal focus and the mirror. In that case the reflected rays will still be diverging (Lesson No. 3 Fig. 8) and will never come to a focus. We can only find a NEGATIVE focus by tracing the rays back to the point from which they appear to have come, behind the glass. Answer: The image will be virtual, upright, enlarged and behind the mirror. (*Rule 36* and Lesson No. 3 Fig. 11.)

53. In this case the object is between the principal focus and center of curvature. Therefore the image will be beyond the center of curvature, real, inverted and enlarged. (*Rule 34.*)

54. The point which I wished to bring out in this question was the fact that no object is so small but it will extend above or below the point called the center of curvature. If the object were simply a point, the rays would all come back to the place from which they started, but as it extends above and below the center of curvature only that part that lies directly upon the center will come under this law. The remaining parts of the object, not being situated upon the center of curvature will be reflected according to the laws which govern Secondary Axes. Rays from above the center will be reflected to the other side of the perpendicular and come to a focus below the center. Rays which leave the object below the center will be reflected to the other side of the perpendicular and come to a focus above the center. Hence the image will be inverted.

55. There are only two kinds of image, real and virtual. Either of these may be produced by a concave mirror according to the location of the object. You have probably noticed by this time that real images are always inverted and that virtual images are always upright.

56. Between the center of curvature and principal focus. (*Rule 34.*)

57. Between the principal focus and the mirror. (*Rule 36.*)

58. At the center of curvature. (*Rule 33.*)

59. Against the glass. (*Rule 36.*)

60. Fully covered in Rules 37 and 38 and diagrams 12 and 13 in Lesson No. 3.

61. A Cylindrical mirror is one which is curved in one direction and straight in the other. If you will take a length of stove-pipe and split it in two lengthways, one of the halves would represent a cylindrical mirror. If you will set it on edge and look towards the concave side, the surface will be exactly the same as a concave cylindrical mirror. On the other side the surface would represent a convex cylindrical mirror. The straight portion is called the axis of the mirror, while the curve is at right angles to it. The axis is precisely like a plane mirror, making the image the same size as the object. The curve acts exactly as any concave or convex mirror would. If you stand this mirror with its axis vertical and look into the concave side, your height will remain the same, but your width will be smaller, making you appear very tall and slim. If you will turn it on its side so that the axis is horizontal you will appear very short and wide because the width is uneffected, while the height is materially decreased. To obtain the image as described in the question, we would have to use a concave cylindrical mirror with its axis horizontal and stand beyond the center of curvature. This will give us a short inverted image, but with the width unchanged. Hence you will appear very short, very wide and up-side down.

62. Only when perpendicular. (*Rule 39*).   63. Toward the perpendicular. (*Rule 40.*) 64. From the perpendicular. (*Rule 41.*)

65. Index really means a sign or symbol. Index of Refraction therefore means a sign or figure which represents the refractive power of a given substance. Thus the index of refraction of air is the figure 1. Of water it is the figure 1.3, and so on. Answer: It is a number or figure used to tell us how many times more than air a given substance can refract, or bend, light.

66.–67. Exactly the same answer applies to both of these—make the ray strike more obliquely. (*Rule 43.*)

68. Exactly the same direction that it had before entering but each ray will be slightly displaced to one side.

69. Every ray will be bent toward the base or thick edge of the prism.   70. As each ray will be refracted alike they will still be parallel and therefore still a beam.   71. At the posterior principal focus (Lesson No. 4, Fig. 7.)   72. At the anterior principal focus (Lesson No. 4, Fig. 8.)

73. The nearer the object approaches the surface on one side the farther away its conjugate moves on the other side, until the object reaches the principal focus when the rays pass off parallel and there is no longer a focus formed.

73. The nearer the object approaches the surface on one side the farther away its conjugate moves on the other side, until the object reaches the principal focus when the rays pass off parallel and there is no longer a focus formed.

74. They will emerge parallel. (Lesson No. 4, Fig. 7 and *Rule 29.*)

75. Wherever the object is placed the emergent rays will be diverging and never meet. Hence all foci are negative and situated between the object and the surface. (Lesson No. 4, Fig. 9 and 10.)

—————————o◯o—————————

A few of the class sent answers to the first two lessons last week and a number have written to know if they should do so. With the exception of the final examination at the close of the course, do not send in any answers as it will be better to keep them there and compare them with the weekly explanations when they arrive. I have looked over such answers as came in however, and am pleased to note that without exception they show earnest, careful study. As my mail is very heavy I take this means of answering the inquiries that I have received and trust that it will be accepted in the spirit intended—as a courteous reply to your letters.

Sincerely,

DR. H. A. THOMSON.

LESSON NO. 5.

Refraction by Lenses.

THUS FAR IN considering refraction by curved surfaces we have supposed the rarer medium to be situated on one side of the surface, and the denser medium to extend back to an indefinite distance on the opposite side. In refraction by lenses however, the light soon passes through the dense substance and emerges again into the air. We will have then, two refracting surfaces under consideration, one at the point of entrance and the other at the point of emergence. These two surfaces may be both curved surfaces or one may be curved and the other plane. Hartridge, Fig. 12 shows the different forms of lenses, number 1, 2 and 3 being examples of convex lenses while 4, 5 and 6 represent concave lenses. A good practical distinction between convex and concave lenses is that convex lenses are always thickest at the center while concave lenses are thickest at the edge.

We learned in Lesson No. 4, Rule 44, that rays passing through a prism are always refracted toward the base. Fig. 1 represents two prisms of equal size with their bases placed together. If two parallel rays of light AB and CD come in contact with these

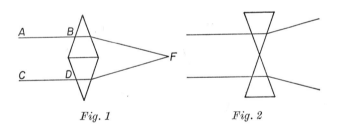

Fig. 1   Fig. 2

prisms at B and D, each will be refracted toward the base and they will cross one another at F thus making a focus for the two rays. As a curved surface is made up of an infinite number of plane surfaces regularly inclined toward one another we may consider lenses to be made up of sections of an infinite number of prisms regularly increasing in strength, the bases being placed together in the convex lens and the angles together in the concave lens. In considering lenses it will only be necessary to consider the action of the bi-convex and the bi-concave lenses since the action of the other forms of convex and concave lenses upon light is identical with these. That is, the plane-convex or the periscoptic convex (converging mensiscus) will bend the rays in the same direction as the bi-convex lens, and the different forms of concave lenses will also be identical with one another in their final action upon the rays.

If a prism always refracts light toward its base, and a convex lens is similar to two prisms placed with their bases together, parallel rays of light passing through it will be refracted toward the center or thickest portion of the lens thus forming a focus at some point behind the lens. If a concave lens is similar to two prisms placed with the apex (angle) of each together, parallel rays passing through it will be refracted away from the center, toward the edges or thickest parts of the lens, and will therefore leave the lens diverging as shown in Fig. 2. We can therefore deduct the following rule, which, if you will constantly keep it in mind, will make the study of refraction by lenses very simple and uncomplicated. Make this heading in your notebook: "Lenses," then copy:

 45. Light passing through a lens, if refracted, is always refracted toward its
  thickest portion.

The principal axis of a lens is a straight line drawn through the centers of curvature of the two curved sutraces. A, Fig. 3, represents the center of curvature of the right surface of the lens CD, and B that of the left surface. The point E, where the principal

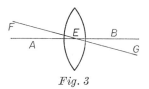

Fig. 3

axis passes through the lens is called the optical center of the lens. In case of a lens having one plane surface, the principal axis is found by drawing a straight line through the one center of curvature and perpendicular to the plane surface. It is evident that a ray of light passing along the principal axis will not be refracted, as it will both enter the lens and emerge from it perpendicular to the surfaces. It was for this reason that I inserted the words "if refracted" in Rule 45, for you will readily see that in the concave lens the axis runs through its thinnest portion and is not bent toward either edge.

Any other straight line as FG Fig. 3 running through the optical center of a lens is called its "Secondary Axis." A ray of light passing along any secondary axis of a lens will be slightly displaced, but will continue in the same direction, as shown in Hartridge, Fig. 13. This displacement is so slight, however, that in ordinary lenses the ray may practically be said to continue straight through the lens without reflection.

If parallel rays of light AD, BE and CF (Hartridge, Fig. 14) come in contact with the convex lens L, the ray BE being upon the principal axis will pass straight through toward H without undergoing any refraction. The ray AD, striking the first surface of the lens at D will be refracted, according to Rule 40, toward the perpendicular MK, and will then continue in a straight line until it reaches the second surface when, according to Rule 41, it will be refracted from the perpendicular NO, taking the direction OH. The ray CF will, in the same manner, be refracted toward H, thus forming a focus of the rays at H. The rays having been originally parallel, this will of course be called the principal focus, and as in the case of the concave mirror, we will call the distance of the principal focus from the lens, the focal length of the lens. If we place our luminous point at the principal focus H the rays diverging from it would pass through the lens and take the parallel directions DA, EB and FC (Rule 29). If parallel rays approach the lens from the opposite side (toward H), they will come to a focus upon the anterior side of the lens at the same distance from the lens as H. We therefore have two principal foci, the anterior and the posterior.

If the rays come from a finite distance in front of the lens, they will be diverging and will come to a focus at some point on the principal axis, farther back than the principal focus, thus forming a conjugate focus of the point at which the light is situated. As we continue to advance the light in the direction of the lens, the conjugate upon the other side will recede from the lens. If we place the light at just twice the focal distance from the lens, we will find its conjugate situated at just the same distance upon the other side. These two points are called "Secondary Foci" and are of great importance to us in the study of lenses. You will find as we proceed that these points take the same part in their relations to the convex lens as the center of curvature does to the concave mirror. It will be well therefore to make a note of them in the notebook. Copy:

46. *The secondary foci of a convex lens are two conjugate foci situated at an equal
      distance each side of the lens at twice its focal length.*

If we place the light at the anterior principal focus, the rays will pass out of the lens parallel. If we place it between the principal focus and the lens, the rays will be so diverging that the lens is not able to entirely overcome them and they will pass out of the lens still diverging, but not so much so as before. There will therefore be no real focus formed, so we can only trace the rays back to the point from which they appear to have come. This point is called a negative focus and is situated upon the same side, but farther back from the lens than the object. If you will draw a picture of a convex lens with the principal axis running through it, as shown at A Fig. 4, and then cut a piece of cardboard in the shape of B Fig. 4, you can very prettily demonstrate these

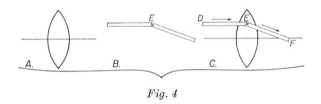

Fig. 4

changes in the position of the different foci. By putting a pin through the hole E and pinning the card to the lens as shown at C, you can let the arm DE of the card represent the incident ray and the arm EF the refracted ray. If placed in the position shown by the diagram, the rays are supposed to be parallel and the arm EF will cross the axis at the principal focus. As a lense will always refract rays striking a certain point of its surface just a certain amount, the angle of the bent ray will be always the same. If we wish therefore to represent the rays coming from a finite distance, we have only to pull down the arm DE until it crosses the axis at the point where the object is supposed to be placed, and the arm EF will cross the axis on the opposite side of the lens at the conjugate focus. You will notice that when the arm DE crosses the axis at just twice the focal distance from the lens, the arm EF will cross upon the other side at just twice the focal distance, thus proving the secondary foci. It will take you but a moment to arrange such a contrivance, and it will richly repay you for the trouble. Try placing the object at every conceivable place and watch the conjugates at each change, and you will soon master this subject.

Images Formed by a Convex Lens.

Having learned to find the focus for any given point, we can easily find the foci for a number of points. Let the arrow AB Fig. 5, represent an object placed at a certain distance from the lens, beyond the anterior principal focus F, and let the line JK repre-

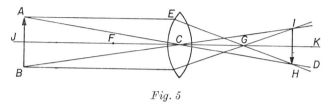

Fig. 5

sent the principal axis. The point A is situated upon the secondary axis AD and will have its focus somewhere on that line. As all rays leaving A will meet after refraction at the same point, it will only be necessary to find where one other ray will cross the line AD, in order to locate the focus. Let us take the ray AE which is traveling parallel to the principal axis. We know that all rays parallel to the principal axis, will be refracted in the direction of the posterior principal focus, so we have only to draw our refracted ray through G in order to find its actual direction. This we do, and find that our ray crosses the secondary axis AD at H. This then, is the focus for the point A. By the same method we can find the focus for the point B at I. We will therefore have an inverted real image of AB at HI smaller than the object. The location and size of the image of course varies with the position of the object. The following rules, which you may copy as you study, will cover these changes. Notice particularly, the wonderful resemblance between the action of the convex lens and the concave mirror. In fact the only difference existing, is that the lens carries the light on through and forms images, while the concave mirror throws them back in the opposite direction. The secondary foci of the lens take the place of the center of curvature in every particular, being twice the distance of the principal focus from the lens, and creating an image at the location of its mate, of exactly the same size as the object. When we consider that the mission of both convex lens and concave mirror is to throw rays of light toward one another, we need not wonder that their effects will be so similar. Copy:

47. in a convex lens, if the object is placed at infinity the image will be real, inverted, smaller than the object, and situated at the posterior principal focus.

48. As the object approaches the secondary focus, the image will move toward the posterior secondary focus increasing slightly in size, but still smaller than the object.

49. If the object is placed at the anterior secondary focus, the image will be real, inverted, of the same size as the object, and situated at the posterior secondary focus.

50. As the object approaches the principal focus, the image recedes toward infinity, constantly and rapidly increasing in size until the object reaches the principal focus, when the rays will leave the lens parallel and there will be no image.

If you will take an ordinary convex spectacle lens, (a good strong one will be best), you can easily demonstrate these changes. By using a lighted lamp for your object and experimenting in a rather dark room, you can easily throw a perfect image of the lamp upon a sheet of paper if the paper is held at the proper distance from the lens. You have only to find the focal length of the lens and the rest will be very easy. To do this, hold the lens in such a position that light coming from the objects upon the street will pass through the lens and strike against your sheet of paper. If you are well back into the room where there is not too much other light to diminish the brightness of the image, you will have, by holding the paper at the proper place, a perfect inverted picture of all the objects upon the street. You have only to move your paper forward and backward a little in order to find the exact focus. As the objects are at a distance of twenty feet or more, this image is at the principal focus, and you have only to measure the distance from your paper to the lens to get the focal length of the lens. You can then proceed to make your experiments with the lens and lamp very accurately, and the changes in size and position of the images will be very impressive and instructive.

Hartridge, Fig. 22, shows very nicely the enlarged, virtual, upright image created by the convex lens when the object is placed between the principal focus and the lens. This is the principle of the watchmaker's eye-glass, or of any magnifying glass, the object being placed inside the principal focus, thus causing the rays to leave the lens diverging and producing a virtual image on the same side of the glass as the object, but farther back and larger. The concave mirror also, as you remember, produces an enlarged, virtual upright image, when the object is placed nearer than the principal focus. Copy:

51. *If the object is placed between the principal focus and the lens, the image will be virtual, upright, enlarged and situated on the same side as the object but farther back from the lens.*

52. *As the object continues to approach the lens, the virtual image also approaches the lens, constantly decreasing in size until the object reaches the lens, when the object and image are of the same size and at the same place.*

Concave Lenses.

In concave lenses a ray from infinity as AD, Hartridge Fig. 19, will strike the lens at D. According to Rule 40 it will be refracted toward the perpendicular CH, and will then continue straight until it reaches the opposite surface when according to Rule 41 it will be refracted from the perpendicular PO, and will take the direction KM. In the same manner the ray CF will be refracted outward. The ray BE being upon the axis passes through without refraction. This gives us diverging rays which, if continued backward to the point from which they appear to have come, give us a "Negative Principal Focus." Diverging rays from a finite distance will be rendered more diverging by the lens, so that we will still have a negative focus, but closer to lens than before.

What is true of one point will be equally true of many points. If we place a candle in front of a concave lens, as AB (Hartridge Fig. 23), we will find the negative focus for the point A situated at "a" and that for B situated at "b." We have then an upright, virtual image of AB at "ab," smaller than the object and situated in front of the lens between the principal focus and the lens. The following rules will cover the conditions arising in the concave lens. Copy:

53. *The image formed by a concave lens is always virtual, upright, and situated in front of the lens, but never farther away than the principal focus.*

54. The image is always smaller than the object except when the object touches the lens, at which time object and image are of the same size and at the same place.

By comparing these two rules with Rules 37 and 38, you will see that the concave lens resembles the convex mirror in its effects upon light, as closely as the convex lens resembles the concave mirror.

Spherical Aberration.

The laws of reflection and refraction by spherical surfaces which we have studied during the past few weeks, are not perfectly accurate unless our mirrors and lenses are only small portions of the spheres. We have said that these spherical surfaces would throw all the rays of light to a single point or focus. This is not strictly true however, for a spherical surface is not the ideal surface for bringing rays to a single point. Fig. 6 will explain this. The rays AB and CD come to a focus at a certain point, while the rays EF

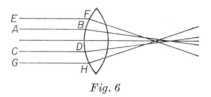

Fig. 6

and GH will come to a point a slight distance in front of that focus. Each succeeding pair of rays then, from the principal axis toward the edge of the lens, will have its focus just in front of the preceding one, so that instead of a focal point we really have a focal line along the principal axis. You can readily see then, that should the lens include a very large portion of the spherical surface the images formed by them would be more or less indistinct. This imperfection in the refractive work of spherical surfaces is called "Spherical Aberration." It is aberration which causes the shadow of a heart to be thrown in the center of a gold ring, when the ring is laid upon a white card and placed in the sun. Spectacle lenses however, as well as lenses for our ordinary optical instruments, are made of such small segments of the entire sphere, that all rays of light passing through them, practically meet at a single focal point, so that except in the case of very strong numbers, the aberration does not interfere in the least with our calculations.

Chromatic Aberration.

If a beam of sun-light be passed through a strong prism, the rays will be unequally divided and will form upon the wall a colored image of the sun which is called the "Solar Spectrum." This image will be found to consist of seven colors in the following order: Red, Orange, Yellow, Green, Blue, Indigo, Violet. White light, then, is made up of seven colors, the violet undergoing the greatest refraction, and the red the least. It is the dispersing of these colors caused by the sun-light shining through drops of rain which produces the rainbow. As lenses are really made up of a number of small prisms they will have the same tendency to disperse colors as the prisms, and the stronger the lens, the greater is this tendency. In the convex lens the violet rays being most refracted will come to a focus nearer the lens than the red rays which are the least refracted. If we hold a screen a little nearer to the lens than these foci, our image will be fringed with red; if we place the screen a little beyond the foci, the rays will have crossed and our image is now fringed with violet. This imperfection in creating a perfect focus is called "Chromatic Aberration."

Some substances disperse light much more than others. Flint glass has a dispersive power nearly twice as great as crown glass. It is important then that spectacle lenses be manufactured from material which has as little dispersive power as possible. The lenses in powerful telescopes and surveyor's instruments are made of a combination of two materials of unequal dispersive power, the one neutralizing the other so that they are entirely free from chromatic aberration. Such a lens is called "Achromatic."

This lesson ends the series on Physical Optics. The different optical instruments built for various purposes are all based upon the laws which we have considered, and are only combinations in different ways of mirrors and lenses. Telescopes, opera-glasses, magnifyers, magic-lanterns, cameras, and hundreds of others, are all based upon these principles. The study of optical instruments and of chromatics is rich with interest and knowledge, and the student is always repaid a hundred-fold for his investigations. We have not space or time however in this course to consider these subjects and must leave them with only the passing glance which we have directed toward them. If the series has been instrumental in creating an interest in this most entertaining science, and a desire for a more thorough knowledge of these subjects, I shall feel more than repaid for my efforts.

For your study between mails begin at Chapter 2 in your Hartridge, and study to "Accommodation" on Page 32. Do not simply read over these pages, but study them, over and over, until they are perfectly understood.

(*End of Lesson No. 5.*)

QUESTIONS ON LESSON NO. 5.

76. If an object is placed one foot from a convex lens whose focal length is 6 inches, where will the image be?
77. If the object is placed 8 inches from the same lens, tell me about the size and location of the image.
78. If the object is placed 4 inches from the lens.
79. If the object is placed against the lens tell me all about the image.
80. If the object is gradually withdrawn from the lens tell me what changes will take place in the image regarding change of size and location, until the object reaches infinity. Answer fully.
81. If the object is placed at the posterior principal focus, where will the image be?
82. How many kinds of images are formed by convex lenses, and what are they?
83. What are the secondary foci of a convex lens?
84. With a convex lens where will you place the object to get a virtual image of the same size as the object?

85. To get a real image the same size as the object?

86. Which of the two images will be inverted, the real or the virtual?

87. Tell me all about the images produced as you gradually draw an object away from a concave lens until the object reaches infinity, giving changes in size, position, etc.

88. If an object is placed at the principal focus of a convex lens, and at some distance from the lens upon the opposite side a concave mirror be placed facing the lens, will there be an image formed? If so, where?

89. If in the place of the concave mirror we put another convex lens, where will the image be?

90. What is your understanding of Spherical Aberration?

91. Of Chromatic Aberration?

LESSON NO. 6.

The Eye.

IF A SMALL opening be made in the end of a dark box, and a convex lens having a focal distance equal to the length of the box, inserted therein, rays of light coming from a distance of twenty feet or more will pass through the lens and form upon the opposite end of the box a perfect inverted, real image of the objects from which the rays proceeded. By making a small peep-hole in the front end of the box, sufficiently distant from the lens so that your head will not obstruct the entering rays, this image can be seen very distinctly.

This is the principle upon which the artist's camera is constructed, the posterior end of the box being removed and a ground-glass slide inserted in its place so that by covering the instrument and his head with a black felt cloth, to shut out the surrounding light, the artist can view the image at his leisure, and can adjust the instrument so as to obtain the most distinct and perfect picture. When every thing is ready he quickly inserts a chemically prepared glass plate, directly in front of the ground-glass, and the image received upon this plate produces certain effects upon the chemicals, resulting in a permanent picture, from which as many photographs as you desire may be copied.

The eye is a most perfectly constructed optical instrument, built upon the same optical principles as the artist's camera, but many times more perfect in its action. It consists of a dark box, or chamber, with a transparent convex surface at the front; a small opening to admit the light; a perfect convex lens placed just behind the opening; and a highly sensitive membrane forming the inner lining of the back wall. Light entering the eye is first refracted to a certain extent by the convex transparent surface, passes in through the small opening and on through the convex lens which again refracts it, forming a perfect image upon the membrane. This membrane consisting of a network of sensitive nerves, is conscious of every disturbance created by the light striking against it, and this sensation being transmitted along the optic nerve to the brain constitutes vision.

The human eye is nearly spherical in shape and about one inch in diameter. It is made up of three walls or enveloping coats and contains three fluids, or humors. The outer coat, or white of the eye, is called the "Sclerotic," and is a tough, strong membrane which serves to maintain the shape of the eye. It is an opaque membrane thus keeping the interior of the eye dark, except at the anterior portion, where it becomes perfectly transparent to allow rays from the object looked at, to enter the eye. This transparent portion which is more convex than the balance of the eyeball, is set into the sclerotic coat precisely like a watch glass and is known as the "Cornea." If you will have your friend stand between yourself and the window with his side turned toward you, you can readily see the cornea by looking across his eye toward the light. You will see that it stands out from the eye, is perfectly transparent, and as stated before, has the same appearance as a watch glass.

The next coat with which we come in contact as we cut through the sclerotic, is the "Choroid." This membrane contains the arteries, veins and vessels which nourish the eye, and on the inner side is covered with a dark, velvety substance known as the black pigment. The office of this pigment is to destroy or absorb the rays of light as soon as they have done their work of forming the image. Were it not for this, the light would be reflected from one side to the other of the eye, creating a sensation at each contact, thus completely dazzling and lighting up the interior of the eye. It is the absence of this pigment in the Albino which makes his eyes so sensitive to light and renders vision almost intolerable.

The third, or inner lining of the eye, is the "Retina." It is upon this membrane that the image of outside objects is formed. It is made up of a complete network of nerves, and is simply a continuation of the Optic Nerve which enters the eye at the back, a short distance to the nasal side (side toward the nose) of the center. The optic nerve is made up of a bundle of tiny nerves, of an infinite number, encased in a membrane or sheath, just as a cable of telegraph wires are wrapped in a rubber casing. This bundle of nerves penetrating into the eye, is spread out upon the inner surface, thus forming the Retina. At every point of the retina are located the ends of some of these nerves, each conveying its own story independently to the brain.

Two points of special interest are present upon the retina, viz.: The Macula Lutea, or yellow spot, and the Optic Disc, or blind spot. The former is situated directly in the path of the entering rays and constitutes the point of direct vision. As you turn your eyes to look from one object to another you simply move this portion of the retina into position to receive the rays of light. As you look across the room at some particular object, as a door-knob, you see that object very distinctly, but are also conscious of the presence of other objects about the room, as pictures, chairs, tables etc. but if you wish to see these objects clearly you must turn your eyes from the direction of the door-knob toward each object successively. The reason for this is easy to understand. The region of the mucula contains a great many more nerve points, and is therefore much more sensitive to light than any other portion of the retina. As you look toward the door-knob the rays proceeding from it enter the eye and form a focus upon the yellow spot enabling you to see the knob very distinctly. Rays from other objects enter the eye upon secondary axes and form their images at different points upon the retina, at a greater or less distance from the yellow spot and are therefore seen, but not so distinctly as the knob. The retina decreases in sensitiveness from the yellow spot outward. As you look upon a printed page an image of the page is formed upon the retina, covering the yellow spot and extending a considerable distance each side. Only the yellow spot however is sufficiently sensitive to distinguish the forms of letters, so that you only see one word at a time together with perhaps a letter or two in the first lines above and below the one you are looking at. Beyond this the page is only a confused mass of letters owing to these other portions of the retina lacking sufficient sensibility to distinguish the outline of such small objects as letters.

The Optic Disc, or blind spot, is that portion of the retina where the optic nerve enters the eye together with the arteries and veins which supply the eye with nourishment. At this spot no nerve fibers are present and rays of light falling upon it create no sensation whatever. This may be very easily demonstrated. Hold this paper about a foot from your face, cover the left eye, and look with the right directly at the cross in Fig. 1. At the same time you will be conscious of the presence of the black dot at the

Fig. 1

right of where you are looking. Now slowly move the paper nearer and farther from your face, always keeping your eye upon the cross, and you will find that at one position the black dot will entirely disappear, leaving the paper of an unbroken whiteness. This is only because the rays from the black dot are now falling upon the Optic Disc and therefore produce no sensation. If you draw the paper a little nearer, the black spot will again appear in view; carry the paper back and it once more disappears; and if you still continue to withdraw the paper, the spot again becomes visible. The reason that the blind spot is not an inconvenience to us in vision, is because rays from an object never fall upon this spot in both eyes at the same time, but are always received upon the sensitive portion of at least one of the retinae.

The three fluids or humors of the eye are the "Aqueous Humor" the "Vitreous Humor" and the "Crystalline Lens." As we enter the eye through the Cornea we first come to the aqueous humor which is, as it's name implies, only water. This humor serves to fill out and hold in shape the cornea and the anterior portion of the eye-ball. Passing through the Aqueous Humor and on through the pupil, we next meet with the Crystalline Lens which, with the muscle and tendon which holds it in place, forms a complete partition across the eye, thus constituting a back wall to the anterior portion of the eye, through which the Aqueous Humor does not penetrate. The Crystalline Lens is a perfect bi-convex lens, slightly more convex at the back than front, is clear as crystal, and so perfectly constructed that Spherical and Chromatic Abberration are almost entirely overcome. Cataract is a disease of this lens by which it gradually becomes more and more opaque until it is impossible for light to penetrate through it. The expression used by many people that a certain person has a cataract "growing over his eye" is, as you will see, an absurd one, as the changes are taking place within the eye and not upon its anterior surface. The only cure for this condition is the removal of the entire lens by the surgeon, after which another lens of equal power must be substituted in a spectacle frame. Behind the Crystalline Lens, and occupying the entire cavity between the lens and the retina, is the "Vitreous Humor." This Humor is a jelly-like substance, firm and elastic in its composition, and as clear as a piece of ice. It serves to maintain the tension and solidity of the eye, which would otherwise collapse upon the slightest pressure.

In the anterior portion of the eye-ball, directly in front of the crystalline lens hangs a circular flexible curtain called the "Iris." This constitutes what we call the color of the eye, the color varying in different individuals, from a deep black to light blue or gray. In the center of this curtain is a round hole, or aperture through which the light passes on its way to the retina. This aperture, called the "Pupil," appears like a black spot to the observer, but only because the interior of the eye is dark. Glance at the house across the street and you will see that the windows appear black, owing to the interior of the building being darker than the outside daylight. The mission of this

Iris is to shut out all unneccessary light and thus keep the eye dark within. In the case of our dark box, if the front end should be removed the picture produced by the lens upon the back wall would be very indistinct, owing to so much light entering the box and thus lighting up the interior. It is so with the eye. The owl has a very large pupil which permits him to gather in a great many rays so that in the dark he is enabled to bring all the feeble scattering rays to a focus upon his retina, thus forming a very distinct image of the surrounding objects. In the daylight however, so much light enters through his large pupils that the eye is dazzled and he can with difficulty find his way from one place to another. The pupil of the human eye is, to a considerable extent, adjustable so that in a bright light it contracts and becomes very small, while in the dark it dilates very strongly, thus regulating at all times the supply of light entering the eye. It is owing to an extensive range of adjustment in the cat's eye which enables him to see almost equally as well by night as day. During the day his pupil appears as a very narrow slit, while at night it becomes round and as large in proportion to the size of his eye as the owl's. The Iris floats in the Aqueous Humor and divides the space occupied by that Humor into two compartments, or chambers. The space between the Iris and the Cornea is given the name of "Anterior Chamber"; that between the Iris and Lens being called the "Posterior Chamber."

Entirely surrounding the lens and attached to it by means of the tendons which hold the lens in place, is the "Cilliary Muscle," its outer edge being attached to the walls of the eye. The work and uses of this muscle are of so much importance in our studies that a consideration of its action will be reserved for another lesson.

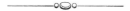

An organ of so much importance and of such delicate adjustment should certainly be placed in a position of safety. Nature has not neglected the care and protection of this little instrument but has placed around it many means of protecting it from accident or injury. It is placed deeply in the head, surrounded on all sides save the front by a bony wall, so that it is difficult for any external object to come in contact with the eye, without being interrupted by these walls. The eye-ball is imbedded in a cushion of oily fat making it as easy for the eye to turn about as though it floated in water. The eye-brow act like a thatched roof in turning aside the perspiration which would otherwise trickle from the forehead into the eyes. The eye-lids serve as a covering to the eye and by constantly wiping the eye-ball keep it moist and bright. At night these lids serve as a covering to the eye while we sleep, the eye at the same time turning slightly upwards, so that should any external substance strike the face during sleep the cornea would escape injury. The lashes which line the margins of the lids, are extremely sensitive to the touch, and immediately close against the entrance of insects or particles of dust or dirt. The eye ball is kept constantly lubricated by the secretion of tears, which, after flowing over it, are passed along through the nasal duct to the nose.

The movements of the eye are controlled by six muscles. These are divided into two classes, the four "Recti Muscles" and the two "Oblique Muscles." The Recti, or straight, muscles are attached to the extreme back wall of the orbit, or bony cavity which contains the eye. From this point of attachment they gradually separate from one another, attaching themselves to the eye-ball at four different points, one at the top, one at the bottom and one at each side. The names given to these Recti Muscles are "Superior" (the upper), "Inferior" (the lower), "External" (the one attached to the temporal side) and "Internal" (the one attached to the nasal side). If you will imagine a large globe, turning upon its center, and fastened at its four sides by long ropes extending back across the room to your hand, and will consider how you must handle these ropes in order to control the different movements of the globe, you will readily understand the action of the Recti Muscles. The Superior Rectus turns the eye upward; the Inferior, downward; the External, outward toward the temple; and the Internal, toward the nose. If it is desired to turn the eye upward and outward at the same time, the Superior and External Recti must act simultaneously. To look downward and outward the Inferior and External act together; upward and in, the Superior and Internal; downward and in, the Inferior and Internal. With the two eyes together if it is desired to glance to the left, the External Rectus of the left eye, and the Internal Rectus of the right are called upon to act. To turn the eyes toward an object held close to the face the Internal Recti of both eyes must work together, and if the object is at the same time held a little above or below the level of the face, the Superior or Inferior Recti must also act in conjunction with the Interni. Again if an object is held a little above and a little to the left, quite close to the face, the Internal Recti must converge the eyes towards one another, the Superior must turn them upward, while the left External and the right Internal (which is already at work maintaining convergence) must turn them to the left. You can easily see that the movements and actions of these muscles which control the eye are the most complicated as well as the most precise of any set of muscles in the human body.

No less important or accurate in their functions are the "Oblique Muscles," whose mission is to always keep the two eyes vertical in relation to one another. To make this more clear, let us imagine a straight line to be tattooed across the cornea of each eye, exactly vertical, from top to bottom. As the eyes look toward a distant object, these two lines are parallel to one another. If from some cause one of the eyes should be called upon to rotate slightly, thus turning the line into an oblique position, the other eye will at once take the same motion and the two lines will again be parallel to each other although they are not now vertical. This movement is controlled by the action of the oblique muscles. To illustrate again, let us suppose a knitting needle to be inserted exactly in the center of the cornea, passed through the pupil and on through the center of the retina. If the needle is held firmly in one position it will now be impossible for the eye to turn either up, down, in or out, thus rendering the recti muscles helpless. The Oblique Muscles, however, are free to act, turning the eye a short distance either way upon the needle, just as a wheel is turned upon its pinion or hub.

The names given to the oblique muscles are "Superior" and "Inferior." The Superior is attached at the back wall, at the same point from which the Recti Muscles originate. Instead of proceeding directly to the eye, however, as in the case of the Recti, it passes along the nasal wall of the orbit until it is just opposite the eye-ball, when it passes through a pulley, or loop of bone, on the nasal wall, turns a complete right angle, and attaches itself to the top of the eye. By contracting this muscle therefore, the upper portion of the eye can be made to turn downward toward the nose. The Inferior Oblique muscle is attached to the lower surface of the eye-ball, extends a short distance toward the nose, and is then attached to the floor of the orbit. The contraction of this muscle turns the lower portion of the eye upward toward the nose, thus turning the upper portion outward from the nose. I trust that the effects of the Oblique Muscles upon the eye have been made clear to you. I notice that many pupils form the idea that these muscles, from their name I suppose, are used to turn the eyes in an oblique direction, for instance upward and outward. This is not so, as such motion is brought about by combined action of the Superior and External Recti. To use a homely expression, the only work of the oblique muscles is to keep the eyes "right side up." The importance of this work is evident. The Retina of the two eyes are an exact counterpart of one another, the nerve ends at any point of one retina being identical with those of the same point of the other. It is therefore always necessary that the images of an object formed by the two eyes, shall fall upon exactly the same portions of the retinae. Should they fail to do so, two separate impressions will be conveyed to the brain and double vision ("Diplopia") is the result. Referring again to our illustration of the globe and ropes, it will be easily seen that were there not some restraining power, the globe could be very easily rolled to one side, out of its upright position and might even be made to turn completely over, thus twisting your ropes and rendering you helpless to give the globe any further adjustment. This necessary restraining power is supplied to the eye in the form of the oblique muscles, which are constantly upon the alert to hold the vertical axes of the two eyes always parallel to one another regardless of the influence which the Recti muscles might otherwise have upon the eye-balls.

Attached to the sclerotic coat and completely encircling the eye a short distance back of the cornea's edge, is the "Conjunctiva." This is a membrane which extends backward a short distance, folds upon itself like a letter V and returning again toward the front is attached at its outer edge to the walls of the orbit. This enveloping membrane serves as a covering to the eyeball, hiding the Recti and Oblique Muscles from view and protecting these muscles as well as the optic nerve from any particles of dirt which might by accident become lodged around the eye. With the Conjunctiva, no foreign substance can possibly work back farther than its fold so that there is no danger of interference with the regular working functions of these muscles and nerves.

The Refraction of the Eye.

Having considered the eye in all its parts and construction, let us now direct it towards a luminous point situated at a distance of twenty feet or more. We have in the eye several refracting surfaces and refracting media, the whole combined constituting what is known as the "Dioptric System of the Eye." In that portion of Hartridge given you for study at the close of Lesson No. 5 this dioptric system is very thoroughly considered together with the cardinal points of the eye, so that it will be unnecessary to repeat what he has already said. Just a word regarding the Nodal Points might make that subject a little more clear. These points are to the eye what the optical center is to the lens, and any ray passing through them whether upon the principal or a secondary axis will practically pass straight in without refraction. The reason of there being two of these points may be understood by a glance at Hartridge Fig. 13. A ray entering upon any secondary axis does not really pass through without refraction but is slightly displaced to one side. If now we will mark upon the principal axis two points, one toward which the entering ray is directed, the other from which the emergent ray appears to have come, we will have the nodal points of that lens. They are situated so closely together however that we practically consider them as one point and call it the optical center. The same is true of the eye. A ray entering upon a secondary axis is displaced from one Nodal Point to the other but so slightly that we can practically consider the two points as one.

For the sake of simplicity we will now consider the dioptric system of the eye as a convex lens, and the Retina as a screen upon which the image is to be formed. Having directed the eye, as already stated, toward a luminous point situated at infinity we will consider the course taken by the rays of light. These rays will of course approach and enter the eye parallel to one another. If the Retina is situated exactly at the principal focus of the dioptric system there will be a perfect inverted image or picture of the luminous point thrown upon the yellow spot, and the point will be distinctly seen. It is always Nature's intention to construct the eye upon this principle, placing the Retina just at the principal focus. Such a condition is given the name of "Emmetropia," or we say that an eye whose principal focus is upon the Retina is an "Emmetropic Eye." Were it possible for nature to accomplish this normal result in all eyes there would be very little need for opticians, but unfortunately a great many eyes are far from Emmetropic, the Retina being placed either too near or too far from the lens, or the lens or cornea may be imperfect in curvature thus forming an imperfect image upon the Retina. To these abnormal, or defective conditions is given the general name of "Ametropia" (the first syllable pronounced like the word "Ah.") Any eye which is not Emmetropic is called "Ametropic."

Ametropia is divided into several classes, according to the different conditions which may exist. Thus if the eye-ball is too long, throwing the Retina back beyond the principal focus, the defect is called "Myopia"; if too short, "Hypermetropia." Hartridge, Fig. 26 and 27, very prettily shows the three conditions of Emmetropia, Hypermetropia, and Myopia. If the eye be a Hypermetropic one and we direct it toward the luminous point as before, the parallel rays will not come to a focus upon the Retina but would focus at some point farther back. The Retina, intercepting this cone of rays on its way to the focus, only succeeds in obtaining a circle of diffused light and therefore gets only a blurred image of the object instead of a distinct one. What can we do to assist this eye in getting a clear image? If the Retina could be carried backward to the correct position the desired object would be attained but this it is impossible to do. If the dioptric system of the eye had a stronger refractive power the principal focus would be nearer to the lens and therefore nearer to the retina. Placing a convex lens before the eye would certainly add to the refractive power by aiding the work of bringing parallel rays to a focus, and if we use a lens of just the right strength the principal focus will be brought exactly to the retina and the eye will be made Emmetropic.

If a Myopic eye be turned toward the luminous point, the parallel rays will be brought to a focus, and will cross and diverge before reaching the retina, thus again forming a diffused circle instead of a distinct point. In this case the refraction of the eye has been too strong thus bringing the rays to a focus sooner than is desired. We have two ways of overcoming this difficulty. One would be to bring the luminous point closer to the eye until its conjugate touched the retina, for we know that as we bring an object closer, the focus gradually moves farther back. The myopic eye then can only obtain a distinct image of objects by bringing them within a limited distance, and the greater amount of myopia (that is, the longer the eye) the nearer must the object be brought. Such an eye is called "Near Sighted" for it can only see distinctly when the object is quite close. The Hypermetropic eye is called "Far Sighted," not because of its ability to see farther than the Emmetropic eye, for we know it cannot, but simply given that name on account of the condition being directly opposite to that of myopia.

The second method of aiding the myopic eye to see the luminous point is, instead of bringing the point nearer, to move the focus upon the retina, the object remaining at infinity. To do this the refractive power of the eye must be lessened. A concave lens of the right strength, from its tendency to bend rays outward instead of together, will, when placed before the eye subtract from its refraction and move the principal focus backward to the retina, thus making the eye Emmetropic. From this subtracting power of concave lenses and adding power of convex lenses, the names minus and plus have been given to them which we shall hereafter use, always calling the concave a minus lens, and the convex a plus lens.

———————o◯o———————

The system of numbering lenses according to their different refractive power is very clearly explained by Hartridge in your last study. A plus lens whose principal focus is one meter (about 40 inches) behind it, or a minus lens whose principal negative focus is one meter in front of it, is called a lens of one dioptre. If the principal focus is one half meter away, the lens must be twice as strong as before, for the stronger the lens the nearer will be the focus. Hence we call it a two dioptre lens one-fourth of a meter (25 centimeters, or ten inches) is the focal distance of a four dioptre lens, and so on. This is a little difficult to understand at first, but if you will bear in mind that "Dioptre" always refers to STRENGTH, or refractive power, while "Meter" and "Centimeter" are applied to FOCAL DISTANCE you will keep these points clear. The focal distance and the refractive strength always vary inversely to each other. That is, to express the focal distance we invert the number which expresses the refractive power. For instance one half dioptre indicates a focal length of two meters; three dioptre one-third meters; five meters, one-fifth dioptre; two thirds of a meter, three halves or one and one-half dioptres written 1.50 D,) and so on. The old method of numbering lenses was to give the lens the number corresponding to its focal length in inches, but for reasons given by Hartridge this system was found in many ways objectionable and the dioptric system was adopted. If at any time however you wish to know the number in dioptres of a lens marked in inches, or vice versa, you can find it by dividing 40 by the given number. Thus 2D equals a 20 inch lens, 4 inch equals 10D.

The summary of this lesson may be condensed into the following notes. Make this heading in your notebook "THE EYE," then Copy:

55. *The Sclerotic is the outer coat or lining of the eye, merging into the cornea at the front and the sheath of the optic nerve at the back.*

56. *The Choroid is the middle wall of the eye containing the blood vessels, and the black absorbing pigment.*

57. *The Retina is the inner lining of the eye consisting of an extension of the optic nerve, and serves as the sensitive screen upon which the image is formed.*

58. *The Optic Nerve extends backward from the eye carrying the retinal sensations to the brain.*

59. *The Optic Disc, Papilla, or Blind Spot is that portion of the retina where the optic nerve enters the eye. This spot is not sensitive to light.*

60. *The Macula Lutea, Fovea Centralis, or Yellow Spot is the point of central vision and is the most sensitive portion of the Retina.*

61. *The Aqueous Humor fills the anterior portion of the eye; the Vitreous Humor the posterior; and the Crystalline Lens and Cilliary Muscle, the space between the two.*

62. *The Iris, or colored portion of the eye, is a circular curtain floating in the aqueous humor, having an aperture at its center called the pupil, and serves to regulate the supply of the light.*

63. *The Cornea is the transparent front of the eye through which the light is first admitted.*

64. *The eye is controlled by four Recti Muscles and two Oblique Muscles. The Recti, called the Superior, Inferior, External and Internal, turn the eye in different directions. The Oblique, called the Superior and Inferior, keep the vertical axes of the two eyes parallel.*

65. *The Conjunctiva is an enveloping membrane which covers the ocular muscles from view and serves as a protection against the entrance of foreign substances.*

66. *The Nodal Points of the eye are two points so situated that if an incident ray is directed toward one of them it will emerge as if coming from the other. Together they constitute the optical center of the eye.*

67. *Emmetropia is that condition of the eye in which the principal focus of the dioptric system is upon the retina.*

68. *Hypermetropia, or Hyperopia, is that condition in which the principal focus is behind the retina.*

69. *Myopia is that condition in which the principal focus is in front of the retina.*

70. *Convex lenses are called plus lenses, concave are called minus.*

71. *The refractive power of a lens varies inversely as its focal distance.*

For your study between mails commence at "Accommodation" on Page 32 ending at "Convergence" on Page 41. I trust you do not neglect these preparation studies. Many of the subjects I have but briefly considered in the lessons owing to the comprehensive explanations given by Hartridge, and if you fail to study these subjects you will certainly be a loser in many ways.

————o◯o————

If you can borrow a copy of "Grays Anatomy" from your physician you will find Diagrams 285 and 530 of great aid to you in studying this Lesson No. 6.

(*End of Lesson No. 6.*)

QUESTIONS ON LESSON NO. 6.

92. How many different substances does light pass through in entering the eye, and what are they?

93. What is Choroid, and what are its uses?

94. Explain the retina fully, naming some of its most important points.

95. What name is given to the outer coating of the eye?

96. What regulates the supply of light entering the eye, and in what manner is it accomplished?

97. What muscles act in turning the eye upward and outward?

98. In turning it downward?

99. Downward and inward?

100. In turning both eyes toward a near object?

101. What other Muscles aid in controlling the eye's movements, and what is their action?

102. What is your understanding of Emmetropia?

103. What other refractive conditions of the eye have you learned? Explain each?

104. What is meant by the word "Ammetropia"?

105. What kind of lens would you use in correcting Hypermetropia?

106. In correcting Myopia?

107. Explain the Dioptric system of numbering lenses?

108. What is the focal distance of a three-fourths dioptre plus lens?

109. What is the dioptric number of a lens whose old style number is 16?

110. Give its focal length in centimeters.

EXPLANATIONS ON LESSONS NO. 5 AND NO. 6.

76. If the principal focus of the lens is 6 inches away then the secondary focus must be one foot away. (*Rule 46.*) Hence the image will be one foot from the lens on the other side. (*Rule 49.*)

77. 8 inches is between 6 inches and 12 inches. Therefore the object is between the principal focus and secondary focus. Hence the image will be beyond the secondary focus on the other side. (*Rules 49 and 50.*)

78. 4 inches is less than 6 inches. Therefore the object is between the principal focus and the lens. Hence the image is on the same side as the lens but farther back. (*Rule 51.*)

79. The image is at the same place. (*Rule 52.*)

80. When object is against the lens, image is virtual, upright, same size as the object and at the same place; when object is between the lens and principal focus, image is virtual, upright, enlarged and farther from the lens; when object is at the principal focus there is no image; when object is between the principal and secondary foci, image is real, inverted, enlarged and beyond the posterior secondary focus; when object is at the anterior secondary focus, image is real, inverted, same size and at the posterior and secondary focus; when object is beyond the secondary focus, image is real, inverted, smaller and between posterior and secondary foci; when object is at infinity, image is real, inverted, very small, and at the posterior principal focus. (*Rules 47 to 52.*)

81. Rays will leave the lens parallel and never meet. (*Rule 50.*)

82. Two, real and virtual, according to the location of the image.

83. A certain pair of conjugates that are situated at an equal distance each side of the lens and at twice the focal length. The principal foci are first, or "principal" in importance. These are "secondary" in importance.

84. Against the lens. (*Rule 52.*)

85. At one of the secondary foci. (*Rule 49.*)

86. Real images are always inverted. Virtual images are always upright.

87. With the object against the lens image is virtual, upright, same size and same place, as object is withdrawn from the lens the image also recedes from the lens, on the same side of the lens, but not so rapidly as the object, and steadily decreases in size. It is still virtual and upright. When the object reaches infinity the image has just reached the principal focus and is very small. (*Rules 53 and 54.*)

88. If the object is on the principal focus on the lens the rays will pass out from the other side of the lens parallel (*Rule 50*) and will continue parallel, just as if they had come from infinity, until they strike concave mirror. Parallel rays striking a concave mirror are thrown to a focus at the principal focus of the mirror. (*Rule 25.*) Hence the image will be at the principal focus of the concave mirror.

89. If we put a convex lens in the place formerly occupied by the concave mirror it will catch the rays that are coming parallel from the first lens and throw them to a focus at its principal focus. (*Rule 47.*) Hence the image will be at the posterior principal focus of the second lens.

90. It is an imperfection of focus caused by spherical surfaces. Instead of all rays meeting at one point those passing through the outer edges are more strongly refracted than those passing through the more central portions.

91. It is an imperfection of focus caused by different colored rays being unequally refracted. It is this imperfection that causes a rainbow colored fringe to appear on white objects when looked at through a cheap telescope or opera glass.

92. Five. The Cornea, Aqueous Humor, Crystalline Lens, Vitreous Humor and Retina. The retina is a transparent membrane and allows the rays to pass entirely through it into the black pigment behind. It is this piercing of the retina that produces the sensation we call Light.

93. It is the middle coating of the eye-ball. It contains the arteries and veins which nourish the eye and the black absorbing pigment which absorbs the rays the instant they have passed through the retina.

93. It is a thin transparent membrane made up of nerve fibers which are a continuation of the optic nerve. It is spread out over the inside of the eye ball forming the third coat or inner lining Each nerve fiber is susceptible to light waves and tells its own independent story to the brain. The important points are the Macula Lutea, where a large number of nerve fibers are entirely absent.

95. The Sclerotic coat.

96. The Iris and Pupil. In dim light the pupil involuntarily dilates to admit more rays. In strong light it contracts.

97. Superior and External Recti.   98. Inferior Recti.

99. Inferior and Internal Recti.   100. Internal Recti.

101. The Superior and Inferior Oblique Muscles. The Superior pulls the top of the eye over sideways toward the nose. The Inferior pulls the bottom of the eye sideways toward the nose.

102. I suppose most of you said "A normal eye," but such an answer would be incorrect. We may have an eye that is diseased or one that is entirely blind and yet it may be emme-

tropic, and such eyes are certainly not normal. Even a dead man's eye may be emmetropic. Emmetropia is that condition in which the principal focus of the eye is situated exactly upon the retina.

103. Hypermetropia is that condition in which the crystalline lens is too weak for the length of the eye. Myopia is that condition in which the lens is too strong for the length of the eye.

104. That condition in which the principal focus of the eye is not situated upon the retina.   105. A convex, or plus, lens.

106. A concave, or minus, lens.

107. The dioptric system is based upon the REFRACTIVE POWER of the lens instead of its focal length. A lens which can bring rays to a focus at a distance of just one meter is called a 1. D. lens. One which can bring rays to a focus at half that distance must be twice as strong and is called a 2. D. lens, and so on. The focal length decreases as the dioptric power increases.

108. To find the focal length in centimeters of any lens we divide 100 cm by the dioptric power, 100 divided by three-fourths (0.75 D) is one hundred and thirty-three and one-third centimeters.

109. To transpose from one system to the other we divide 40 inches by the given number. 40 divided by 16 gives us 2.50 D.

110. 100 cm divided by 2.50 gives us 40 centimeters, as explained in No. 108.

LESSON NO. 7.

Accommodation.

IF WE PLACE an object at a distance of twenty feet or more before an Emmetropic eye, rays of light from the object will enter the eye parallel and will form an inverted image of the object upon the retina, thus producing distinct vision. If we now move the object closer to the eye placing it for instance at two meters distance, the rays instead of being parallel will be diverging, and the conjugate focus having moved farther back from the principal focus, will be behind the retina. How is it then that distinct vision for objects at a finite distance can be obtained? We know that it is obtained, for you are even now holding this lesson at a distance of less than one meter, still every line is read clearly and distinctly. Had the eye the power to adjust the position of its retina moving it backward and forward as occasion demands, we could readily see that distinct vision for all distances would be maintained.

It was for many years believed that the eye had this power and the question of adjustment for different distances was explained on that line, but it was finally proved that the retina is permanent and immovable and that such a change of position is impossible. That theory proving untrue, the question once more arises, what can be done to bring the image of near objects upon the retina? As in the case of Hypermetropia, if the refraction of the eye could be increased the focus would be moved forward from behind the retina until it once more rested upon the retina. A convex lens placed before the eye would accomplish this result, but we know that the eye has the power of adjusting itself to different distances without this artificial aid. The only remaining explanation is that the crystalline lens must have some means of changing its refractive power, becoming stronger as the object approaches the eye, and weaker as the object recedes. This is what really takes place, and it is for this work that the Cilliary Muscle is created. The crystalline lens is held in place by strong ligaments which during repose hold the lens in its condition of least refractive power and the eye is adapted for parallel rays of light. As the object is brought nearer, the Cilliary Muscle (which surround the lens very much as a spectacle rim surrounds the glass) contracts, and by loosening the tension of the ligaments, allows the lens from its own elasticity to become more convex and therefore stronger. As we continue to bring the object nearer, the lens continues to increase in convexity, the image all the while remaining upon the retina and the vision of course remaining distinct at all times.

This power of the eye to adjust itself to different distances is called "Accommodation." You can easily prove its existence by the experiment mentioned by Hartridge. Stand before a window a foot or two from the wire netting and look at some object across the street. The object will be seen very distinctly but the screen will be indistinct. Now without moving your eyes fix your attention toward the meshes of the screen through which you were previously looking. The screen will now be very distinct but the object across the way will be indistinct. Look once more at the object and you do not see the screen; back to the screen and the object is once more blurred. Continue this for a few times and you will begin to feel conscious of a movement taking place inside your eye at every change, and very soon a feeling of fatigue will be experienced owing to the unusual labor imposed upon the cilliary muscle, very much as the arm becomes exhausted after continuous contraction and relaxation in working with a saw or heavy hammer. Copy:

72. *Accommodation is that function by which the eye is enabled to adjust itself for different distances, thus obtaining at all times a distinct image upon the retina.*

How much accommodation must an Emmetropic eye use in order to distinctly see an object of one meter (40 inches)? To answer this question let us first consider the Emmetropic eye. When this eye is at rest parallel rays of light coming from a distance of 6 meters or more will focus upon the retina without any exertion on the part of the eye, as shown in Hartridge Fig. 26-A. Now if we move the object to a distance of one meter from the eye there will be two methods of obtaining distinct vision, one by means of a convex lens, the other by means of the accommodation. If we use the convex lens the question is, what strength lens will be required? The eye remaining at rest, nothing but parallel rays can be brought to a focus upon its retina, and in order to obtain parallel rays we must use a lens whose anterior principal focus will be situated at the same point as the object. The object being placed at one meter, a lens having a focal length of one meter will change the diverging rays to parallel rays, and thus give the eye distinct vision. A glance at the diagram will make this more clear. Rays coming from the object O which is just at the anterior principal focus of the lens will emerge from the lens parallel and will enter the eye the same as if they came from infinity. The focal length of the lens being one meter its power is one dioptre.

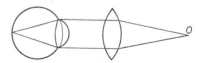

If instead of using a lens of one dioptre to see the object, we let the accommodation do this work, you can easily understand that the refractive power of the eye must be increased just one dioptre in order to attain the same results. The cilliary muscle therefore contracts a sufficient amount to allow the lens to add one dioptre to its original power and we say that the eye has used one dioptre of accommodation. In order to see distinctly at one-half meter (50 centimeters), two dioptres must be used; at one-fourth meter, 4 D; at one-fifth meter, 5 D; at two meters, one-half dioptre, etc. Thus you will see that we can measure the amount of accommodation upon the same principles by which we number our lenses, the accommodation really being represented by a lens whose focal distance is equal to the distance of the object from the eye. If you do not thoroughly understand this stop now and go over it again, for it will be impossible to clearly follow the remainder of the lesson without a perfect understanding of what has just been said. Copy:

73. *The amount of accommodation used by the Emmetropic eye in looking at any*

object, is represented by a convex lens whose focal length is equal to the distance of the object from the eye.

---◦◯◦---

The amount of accommodative power in any eye depends very materially upon the age of the individual. From the age of 10 years this power gradually diminishes through life, until at about 75 the function of accommodation is entirely lost and the eye can only see distinctly at some one given point, that point being at infinity for the emmetropic eye and at some finite distance for the myopic eye. At the age of ten years the accommodation usually amounts to about 14 dioptres; at twenty, 10 D; at thirty 6.50 D (six and one-half dioptres); at forty 4.50 D; at fifty 2.50 D and so on. Copy:

74. *The power of accommodation in any eye gradually diminishes from the age of 10 years, until at about 75 it entirely dissappears.*

In order to determine the amount of accommodation possessed by an eye, two points must be considered, viz.: The far point, or "Punctum Remotum," and the near point, or "Punctum Proximum." The Punctum Remotum is that point for which the eye is adapted when in a perfect state of rest and is of course the most distant point for which the eye can obtain distinct vision. In the emmetropic eye this point lies at infinity, the eye at rest being adapted for parallel rays of light, while in the myopic eye the punctum remotum is situated at some finite distance, for we learned in Lesson No. 6 that in order for the myopic eye to see distinctly the object must be brought nearer than twenty feet until the image formed in the eye moves backward to the retina. The Punctum Proximum is that point for which the eye is adapted when its power of accommodation is exerted to the fullest extent. The nearest point at which the eye can read fine print will be the punctum proximum of that eye. Other methods of determining the punctum proximum are explained by Hartridge in your last study, all based upon the principle of finding the nearest point for which the eye is capable of accommodating. Copy:

75. *The Punctum Remotum is the most distant point for which the eye can obtain distinct vision, being that point for which the eye is adapted when in a state of perfect rest. The refraction of the eye at this time is called the "Statis Refraction" of the eye.*

76. *The Punctum Proximum is the nearest point for which the eye can obtain distinct vision, being that point for which the eye is adapted when exerting its power of accommodation to the utmost. The refraction of the eye at this time is called the "Dynamic Refraction" of the eye.*

Having found both the punctum remotum and punctum proximum of an eye, we can easily determine the amount of accommodation. For instance, the far point of an Emmetropic eye is situated at infinity. If we find that the nearest point at which he can read is one meter from his eye, we know that he has one dioptre of accommodation, for we have already learned that the Emmetrope uses one dioptre of accommodation in looking at an object one meter away. (Rule 73) and as this is his nearest point we know that all of his accommodation has been used. If his near point is at 50 centimeters (one-half meter) his accommodation amounts to 2 D. If at 25 cm (one-fourth meter) he has 4 D of accommodation; at 20 cm, 5 D; at 10 cm, 10 D; at 5 cm, 20 D, etc., one meter being equal to 100 centimeters. If his near point is two meters away he has only one-half dioptre (0.50 D) of accommodation; if at four meters one-fourth dioptre (0.25 D).

The total amount of accommodation found in any eye is called the "Amplitude of Accommodation," and is expressed in dioptres. The distance covered in measuring from the near to the far point is called the "Range of Accommodation." It is necessary that the distinction between these two be perfectly understood, for I find that pupils are very apt to get the two confused, thereby meeting with frequent obstacles in the consideration of this subject. Amplitude of Accommodation simply refers to the power of the lens to become more convex, while Range of Accommodation refers to the territory covered in changing the vision from the far point to the near. Copy:

> 77. *The Amplitude of Accommodation is the accommodative power of the eye*
>   *expressed in dioptres.*
>
> 78. *The Range of Accommodation is the distance between the Punctum Remotum*
>   *and the Punctum Proximum.*

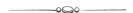

In the Myopic eye the punctum remotum is not situated at infinity but at a finite distance, for parallel rays will come to a focus too soon, thus making it necessary to move the object nearer in order to obtain a clear image upon the retina. The most distant point at which the object can be placed still keeping the focus upon the retina, is of course the far point of vision or punctum remotum.

The punctum proximum, as in the emmetropic eye, is the nearest point at which distinct vision can be maintained. But, with the near points at the same place, will the myopic and emmetropic eyes have the same amplitude of accommodation? For instance let us consider a myope of one dioptre, having his near point at one-half meter, and an emmetrope whose near point is at the same place. We know that the emmetrope's Amplitude of Accommodation is 2 D. But the myope was already adapted for a distance of one meter by virtue of his 1 D of myopia. He will therefore have less distance to cover in changing from one meter to one-half meter, and will consequently use less accommodation than the emmetrope who must change from infinity to one half meter. In other words the emmetrope must use one dioptre of accommodation before he can reach the point for which the myope is already adapted. viz.: one meter. From this point on the two move in unison, each doing the same amount of work until the one-half meter distance is reached, the emmetrope having used 2 D of accommodation, the myope 1 D. The range of accommodation covered by the myope was one-half meter, that of the Emmetrope being all the distance from one-half meter to infinity.

In the Hypermetropic Eye the punctum remotum is neither situated at a finite distance nor at infinity, but is "beyond infinity," for only rays which are converging can focus upon the retina when the eye is in a state of rest. The position of the far point, which is of course negative, is represented by the focal distance of the lens which corrects the hypermetropia. For instance an eye having one dioptre of hypermetropia requires a convex lens of one dioptre to focus parallel rays upon the retina, for when we say that an eye has one dioptre of hypermetropia we simply mean that the refractive power of the dioptric system is one dioptre too weak for the length of the eye, and

it must therefore be increased by the addition of a plus 1 D glass. This glass renders the parallel rays sufficiently converging to enable the eye to bring them together at the macula. These converging rays would have met, had not the eye intercepted them, at just one meter behind the lens. We say therefore that the rays which this eye requires are rays sufficiently converging to have met at one meter behind the eye. This point is called the "Negative Punctum Remotum" of the Hypermetropic Eye. By the same reasoning we find that the negative punctum remotum of an eye which is two dioptres hypermetropic is situated one-half meter behind the eye, and so on. This is perhaps a little difficult to clearly comprehend at first, but if you will remember that in all our considerations of optics, when we do not have a real point or focus, we trace the rays in the opposite direction until they meet, thus creating a negative or imaginary point, I believe that you will understand this negative far point of the hypermetropic eye. In the study of concave lenses, when we found that the refracted rays were leaving the lens diverging, and would therefore never meet at any focal point, we at once turned the other way and found a point from which they appeared to have come, calling it a negative focus. It is the same thing with us here. We know that the converging rays required by the Hypermetrope could never have come from a point, so we turn the other way to find a point at which they might meet, and call it negative.
Copy:

79. The punctum remotum of the Emmetropic eye is situated at infinity.

80. The punctum remotum of a myopic eye is situated at a finite distance, its distance from the eye being represented by the focal length of the correcting glass.

81. The punctum remotum of a hypermetropic eye is a negative one, situated behind the eye at a distance represented by the focal length of the correcting glass.

Both having the same near point will the hypermetropic or emmetropic eye use the most accommodation? Let us consider a hypermetrope of one dioptre, having the punctum proximum at one-half meter before him, and an emmetrope whose punctum proximum is at the same place. The emmetrope's amplitude of accommodation we know to be 2 D. The hypermetrope having a too short eye, must first accommodate one dioptre in order to bring parallel rays to a focus upon his retina and thus place himself upon an equal footing with the emmetrope. From this point on, they must each use 2 D of accommodation, the hypermetrope therefore using a total of 3 D, an excess of 1 D over that of the Emmetrope. It will be clear from the foregoing that a hypermetrope in looking at any given distance must always use an amount of accommodation, equal to the amount of his hypermetropia, MORE than an emmetrope would use in looking at the same point, and that a myope will use an amount of accommodation equal to the amount of his defect, LESS than the emmetrope would use. For instance in the three different eyes which we have considered, viz.: a myope of 1 D hypermetrope of 1 D, and an emmetrope, each having his near point at one-half meter, we find the amplitude of accommodation to be 2 D for the emmetrope, 3 D for the hypermetrope, and 1 D for the myope.

The method of computing the amplitude of accommodation by algebraic formula is so well covered by Hartridge that a repetition would not be necessary. Do not neglect however to study that subject as thoroughly as you do the lesson, for it is equally important.

Let us now consider the solution of a few problems based upon the subjects which we have covered in this lesson.

1st. What is the condition of a person whose Punctum Proximum is at 25 cm (one-fourth meter), and whose amplitude of accommodation is 3 D? In adjusting his eye for an object at a distance of 25 cm we know that the refraction of the eye at that time is 4 D stronger than that of the emmetrope when in a state of rest. As his amplitude of accommodation is 3 D, the eye's refraction when he is not accommodating would still be 1 D stronger than the emmetrope, hence we know that he has a myopia of 1 D.

2nd. Where is the punctum proximum of a person whose amplitude of accommodation is 4 D and whose punctum remotum is situated 50 cm behind his eye? His far point being 50 cm, or one-half meter behind his eye, we know it to be a negative far point, thus proving him to be a hypermetrope of 2 D. As it will require 2 D of his accommodation to correct his hypermetropia and thus place him on an equal footing with and emmetrope, he will have but 2 D remaining with which to approach a near point. 2 D will bring his point of adjustment from infinity to one-half meter (or 50 cm) before him, which is the punctum proximum of his eye.

3d. What is the amplitude of accommodation of a myope of 2 D whose punctum proximum is at 20 cm? An emmetrope would require 5 D of accommodation to adapt himself for this point, but the refractive power of this myopic eye is 2 D stronger than the emmetrope. Hence in approaching a near point the myope has the advantage by that amount and will require but 3 D of accommodation, which is his amplitude of accommodation.

These problems will, I think, be sufficient to give you an idea of this subject and will be a good preparation for the accompanying examination. You cannot drill too thoroughly upon these points as they are the key-note to nearly all that is to follow. For your study between mails finish the second chapter of Hartridge.

(End of Lesson No. 7.)

L E S S O N N O. 7. (Supplement.)

In the first place we must figure everything from the standpoint of the emmetrope. We know that an emmetrope always uses just as much accommodation in looking at a certain distance as the distance is represented in dioptres. Or as many times as the distance in cm is contained in 100. For instance, if an emmetrope looks at a distance of 50 cm in front of him he will use 2 D of accommodation. If he looks at 20 cm in front of him he will use 5 D. Now the emmetrope is the only one who uses just the amount that corresponds to the distance, for the myope uses less and the hypermetrope uses more. If you will get the emmetrope clear in your mind I think you will have no trouble with the others. A hypermetrope always uses more accommodation than an emmetrope, for his eye is shorter and he must make his crystalline lens stronger in order to bring his focus farther forward, so that it will be upon the retina. If he has 3 D of hypermetropia he will have to use 3 D more accommodation than an emmetrope. If he has 5 D of hypermetropia then he must always use 5 D more. For instance if an emmetrope looks at a distance of 33 cm he must use 3 D of accommodation, while if a 2 D hypermetrope looks at the same point he must use 5 D of accommodation. If the emmetrope should look at an infinite distance he would not have to work at all, for that is his resting place, but the hypermetrope must use the 2 D of accommodation even in looking at that distance. If he was a 6 D hypermetrope he would have to use 6 D of accommodation in order to bring his principal focus up to his retina. A myope, on the other hand, has just as much the advantage as the hypermetrope has disadvantage. His eye being longer he does not have to bring his focus so far forward to get to his retina. If he is a myope of 4 D he will use 4 D less accommodation in looking at any point within his range than an emmetrope would use in looking at the same point. If he should have 2 D of myopia he would use 2 D less. If an emmetrope should look at an object at 25 cm he would have to use 4 D of accommodation while if a 3 D myope looks at the same distance he would only have to use 1 D as he has 3 D the advantage. If you will keep this point in your mind you will find it a great help in working out the problems. In fact you can do nothing without it.

There is another point that is very important, and that is that the condition of the eye always tells us where the P. R. is, or if we have the P. R. we can tell the condition of the eye. The eye is always at rest when looking at its P. R. and we can therefore get its exact measure, without the accommodation interfering. We have learned in the lesson that the P. R. of an emmetrope is at infinity. We have also learned that the P. R. of a myopic eye is between the eye and infinity. The distance from the eye tells us just how much of a myope he is. If it is at 50 cm then he is a myope of 2 D. If at 33 cm he is a myope of 3 D, etc. The P. R. of a hypermetrope is always a negative one, and the distance that it is situated back of the eye tells us how much hypermetropia he has. If it is 25 cm behind his eye then he has 4 D of hypermetropia. If 20 cm then he has 5 D and so on. Do not forget this point for in a great many places the question states where the P. R. is, simply to tell you what kind of an eye it is. In other places it tells you what kind of an eye we have simply to enable you to find the P. R. Remember that one always tells the other. It is not so with the P. P. It always tells us the condition of the eye when it is hard at work. In other words when it is working as hard as it possibly can. If you will keep all these points in mind and will remember to compare every single case with an emmetrope I believe that you can handle them all right. Let us take a sample case: Where is the P. R. of an eye whose P. P. is at 20 cm and his amplitude of accommodation is 1 D? Let us see. If his P. P. is at 20 cm that is the place where he is looking when he is at work at his hardest. If he were an emmetrope he would use 5 D of accommodation in looking at this point. As it is he only uses 1 D for that is all that he has and we know that he uses all that he has when he looks at his P. P. If he is seeing at that distance with 1 D of accommodation while an emmetrope would use 5 D he must be a myope of 4 D, for it is only myopes that can reach any near point with less accommodation than an emmetrope. As he uses just 4 D less than an emmetrope he must be a 4 D myope. As stated above the condition tells us the P. R. His condition being myopic 4 D his P. R. will be 25 cm in front of his eye.

Where is the P. P. of an eye whose P. R. is at 1 meter and whose amplitude of accommodation is 4 D? The P. R. of course tells us his condition. As it is situated one meter in front of his eye he must be a myope of 1 D. He has an accommodative power of 4 D. Having 1 D the advantage of an emmetrope he can accomplish as much with his 4 D as an emmetrope could with 5 D. That would bring him to 20 cm, for we know that an emmetrope when using 5 D of accommodation is looking at 20 cm. This can also be solved in another way: We know that his static refraction (measure of his eye at rest) is 1 D myopic. His crystalline lens is too strong for the length of his eye and the rays are focussed before reaching the retina. He has the power to increase the strength of his lens 4 D. That is, when he exerts all his power he can make the lens just 4 D stronger than when he is at rest. If the lens is naturally 1 D too strong he will when at work make it 5 D too strong, hence will make himself temporarily a myope of 5 D. In other words his dynamic refraction (measure of his eye at work) is 5 D myopic. His point of adjustment at that time will of course be at 20 cm, which we call his Punctum Proximum.

I believe that a careful study of the above principles will aid you considerably in determining the answers to Examination No. 7. Always remember to compare each case with the emmetrope and decide from this comparison the condition of the eye under consideration. Do the best you can with the question and if you are still in the dark I will gladly explain further. I realize that this is a hard lesson, but it is as important as it is difficult. Nearly all of the following subjects which we are to take up hinge upon a thorough understanding of the principles involved in Lesson No. 7.

Yours Sincerely,

Dr. H. A. Thomson.

QUESTIONS ON LESSON NO. 7.

111. What is your understanding of accommodation?

112. Explain the physiology of accommodation. That is, explain what action takes place in the eye when accommodating.

113. Are there any people who have no accommodation? If so, why?

114. What name is given to the nearest point at which an eye can see distinctly?

115. What is the state of the eye when looking at that point?

116. What name is given to the most distant point at which the eye can distinctly see, and what is the state of the eye at that time?

117. What is the difference between the Range of Accommodation and the Amplitude of accommodation?

118. Give the location of the punctum remotum in the emmetropic, myopic and hypermetropic eyes.

119. Where is the punctum proximum of an eye whose punctum remotum is 10 cm behind the eye and whose amplitude of accommodation is 14 D?

120. Where is the punctum remotum of an eye whose amplitude of accommodation is 3 D and whose punctum proximum is at 20 cm?

121. If the amplitude of accommodation is 8 D?

122. What is the condition of an eye whose amplitude of accommodation is 4 D and whose punctum proximum is at 25 cm?

123. Where is his punctum remotum?

124. Give the amplitude of accommodation of an eye whose punctum remotum is at two meters and his punctum proximum at one meter.

125. Where is the punctum proximum of an eye whose punctum remotum is 50 cm behind it, and whose amplitude of accommodation is 1 D?

126. Give the amplitude of accommodation of a 2 D myopic eye whose punctum proximum is at 8 cm.

127. Give the range of accommodation of a 3 D myope whose amplitude of accommodation is 3 D.

128. Of a myope of 5 D having the same amplitude of accommodation.

129. State the condition of the eye whose punctum proximum is at 25 cm and whose amplitude of accommodation is 14 D.

130. Where is his Punctum Remotum?

131. Where is the punctum proximum of a one-half dioptre myope 80 years of age?

132. What is the correcting glass for an eye which can read no nearer than 25 cm and whose amplitude of accommodation is 7 D?

133. Give the correcting glass for one whose amplitude of accommodation is 7 D and whose nearest point of distinct vision is 10 cm.

134. For one having 8 D of accommodation and whose punctum proximum is at twelve and one-half centimeters.

135. Give the amount of accommodation necessary to change the adjustment of an eye from three meters to two meters.

136. From one meter to one-half meter.

137. Have you copied all the note-book rules up to date?

LESSON NO. 8.

Convergence.

WHEN THE EMMETROPE directs his attention toward an object one meter in front of him, he is called upon to exert his accommodative power one dioptre to enable him to obtain a distinct image upon his retina. In addition to this work another muscular effort is called forth which must act with a view to placing the yellow spot of each eye in position to receive the image upon each alike. In other words he must turn the eyes in, toward the object, in order to see distinctly with both. This work is carried on by the internal recti muscles and is given the name of "Convergence."

In order to measure the amount of work done in converging for any given point it has been necessary to fix a standard of measurement, and as convergence and accommodation go hand in hand, this standard has been based upon the same principles by which we measure refraction. The force necessary to converge to a distance of one meter is taken as the unit and is called a "Meter-Angle." To turn the eyes toward an object at one-half meter, 2 meter angles of convergence are used, and so on. You will readily see that Nature intends these two functions, accommodation and convergence, to act in harmony with each other, for when the emmetrope is called upon to accommodate 2 D he must also converge 2 M. A; or if he accommodates 3 D he also converges 3 M. A. When looking toward infinity, neither accommodation or convergence is used.

The action of these two functions are so intimately linked together that they can only work independently within certain limits. That is, it is impossible to use the accommodation beyond a certain limit without allowing the convergence to act at the same time, or to converge beyond a certain limit without bringing the accommodation along with it. As an example of the harmonious action of muscles, hold up your hand with the fingers straight. Now close your fingers in the act of doubling your fist. The fingers all close together in unison. Again straighten them and this time try to hold the little finger upright while you crul the others. You will find that to a certain limit this can be done, but beyond that limit the little finger is bound to follow. The Cilliary and Internal Recti Muscles bear this same relation, to one another, so that if one is at any time brought into action, the other will either act or stand ready to act, and beyond a certain limit is bound to act. It is necessary that this harmony between the two muscles be fully understood in order that convergence may be made simple.

To measure the amount of convergence which an eye possesses we must find the strength of the internal recti. One way to do this, would be to have the patient fix his eyes upon an object, and then gradually draw the object nearer to him, until he sees two objects instead of one. At the instant single vision ceases we have reached the limit of his converging powers, and the point reached is the punctum proximum of convergence, from which we can easily determine the amount of convergence. If the nearest point toward which the eyes can converge is at 20 cm the convergence used was 5 M. A. If at 25 cm, 4 M. A., etc. Another method of measuring convergence is by means of prisms. We have learned (Rule 44) that light in passing through a prism is always refracted toward the base. If we place a prism before the right eye with its base out, that is, toward the temple, the rays coming toward the eye will be bent outward by the prism and will appear to the eye as if the object was displaced toward the left, and the eye will of course turn toward the left to receive the impression upon its yellow spot. The eye then in looking through a prism must always turn toward the apex or thinnest portion of the prism in order to receive the rays which are bending toward the base. Copy:

82. The eye in looking through a prism always turns towards the apex.

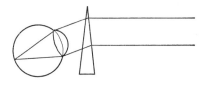

We can then, seat our patient in a chair and direct him to look at a candle or gas flame at a distance of 20 feet. His eyes will of course be parallel and there will be no convergence in use. If we direct him to continue gazing at the flame, and then place a prism before one of his eyes with the base out, that eye must at once turn toward the nose in order to still keep the image upon the retina. He will then, have made an effort of convergence in overcoming the prism. If we continue to add stronger and stronger prisms over one or both of his eyes, still keeping the bases out, the convergence will be regularly increased until the limit is reached. As soon as the strength of the prisms is greater than the power of convergence, the patient will tell you that he sees two flames instead of one, and you will know that his convergence has been used to its utmost capacity. The strongest prism with which he can still see one flame is the measure of his converging power.

The reason why he sees two flames when the prisms are stronger than he can overcome, is very apparent. At each addition of prismatic power the rays are bent more strongly and consequently more to one side of the yellow spot, thus calling upon the convergence to bring the yellow spot once more into place. As we approach the limit of converging power this work becomes more difficult to perform until at length it stops entirely and the next prism throws the image to one side of the yellow spot where it is bound to remain. In that condition we have rays from the flame entering one eye and forming an image upon the yellow spot, and other rays from the same flame entering the other eye, forming an image upon an entirely different portion of the retina, and as the nerves at the yellow spot of the one eye have nothing in common with the nerves of some different portion of the other retina, two separate messages are conveyed to the brain which interprets these sensations as if there were actually two lights.

In the above test with prisms, one point was omitted. That was, the condition of accommodation during the test. We have said that convergence and accommodation move hand in hand, and that they are never separated from one another beyond certain limits. This is as true in this instance as in others. When we direct our patient to look at the flame 20 feet distant he will not, if an emmetrope, use any accommodation. As the prisms refract all parallel rays alike leaving them still parallel, they will have no effect upon the accommodation but will simply influence the convergence. At each increase of prism the convergence will increase accordingly but the accommodation is still held back (though contrary to its tendency), in order to focus the parallel rays upon its retina. This is kept up until the limit is reached, when either the accommodation will begin to exert itself, thus getting a different image of the flame, or, what is more apt to be the case, the convergence will stop and refuse to exert itself further. In that case the stronger prisms simply create double vision ("Diplopia") and the test is at an end unless we can devise some method of overcoming the difficulty. How can it be done? If the accommodation could be induced to act, the convergence would proceed again as before. If a concave lens is placed before an emmetropic eye, the refraction of the eye will be decreased and it will be necessary to use the accommodation in order to bring the refraction up to the correct strength again. In other words the concave glass will make him a hypermetrope, throwing the focus behind the retina and he must accommodate to bring it forward again. This is what we desire, and by placing a pair of minus lenses before the eyes the accommodation is allowed to act, and the harmony between it and convergence is once more restored, so that the test may be continued. This is very interesting work. I have often made this test, adding stronger and stronger prisms until the patient would say that he saw two lights, and could not possibly fuse them into one, when by holding concave lenses before his eyes he would at once exclaim: "Now I see only one light."

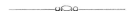

To find the punctum remotum of convergence, or, in other words to measure the diverging power of the eyes, prisms are our only resource. The plan of moving an object farther and farther back would not avail, for we can never reach a point so remote that the rays will not still come to the eyes parallel, and will therefore never induce the eyes to turn outward. By the use of prisms however, we can test the diverging powers very successfully. Requesting the patient to again look toward the flame we begin by placing weak prisms before the eyes (base in this time) continually increasing the strength until diplopia is reached. The strongest prism which he can overcome indicates his power of divergence. The punctum remotum of convergence will of course be a negative one, situated behind the eyes in all cases where there exists any power to diverge, which is almost invariably the rule except in cases of cross-eye ("Internal Strabismus".)

The system of numbering prisms is still in a very imperfect condition, for although it is understood that numbering them by meter-angles is in harmony with the dioptric system it has not as yet been adopted by the manufacturers, or by the profession in general, into their practical work. We are therefore still working by the old system of numbering a prism according to its angle, calling them one degree, two degree, three degree prisms, and so on. While this system is valueless in aiding us to find the exact location of the punctum remotum or punctum proximum without intricate computations, still we can judge of the converging or diverging power of the eyes by the strength of the prism overcome. Hence we say that he has a converging power of 20 degrees, or

30 degrees, as the case may be, or a diverging power of 10 or 12 degrees, and so on. The act of convergence is frequently given the name of "Adduction," that of divergence being called "Abduction." The internal recti muscles are therefore called the "Adducting Muscles," the external, "Abducting Muscles," and prisms placed before the eyes are given the names of "Adducting and Abducting Prisms" according as their bases are placed out or in respectively. The act of turning one eye higher than the other, which is produced by the exertion of the superior rectus of one eye and the inferior rectus of the other, is called "Sursumduction." The sursumducting power is measured by finding the strongest prism which, placed with its base up or down as the case may be, the eyes are capable of overcoming. The average sursumducting power of normal eyes is about 3 degrees, the abducting power usually about 8 degrees, and the adducting power about 40 degrees.

In speaking of these tests I have said that the prisms may be placed before either or both eyes as desired. This might at first thought seem difficult to understand, but we must bear in mind that the only object of the prisms is to turn the eyes closer together or farther apart as the case may be, so that we may accomplish this by placing, say an 8 degree prism before one eye, or a 4 degree prism before each eye. A prism of 6 degrees before one eye and one 2 degrees before the other, also has the same effect. For instance if we are testing the abducting power of the eyes, we might first place a 3 degree prism base in before the left eye, and if diplopia is not produced a 4 degree prism with its base also in, could be placed before the right eye, thus making a total prismatic power of 7 degrees to be overcome. If the 7 degrees should prove too strong, we can reduce the power one degree by either taking off one of the prisms and substituting one which is one degree weaker, or we can leave them alone and place a one degree prism base out before either of the eyes. This prism will neutralize one degree of the 7, leaving now a total of 6 degrees base in, to be overcome. If we are testing the sursumducting power we can place all of the prisms over one eye base up, or over the other base down, or it may be divided into two prisms, one base up before one eye, and the other base down before the other eye, the only object being to determine how much one eye is capable of raising above its fellow. You will readily see that had the patient but one eye, prisms would be of no avail, for the consideration of convergence, divergence, etc., must of course include the action of both eyes.

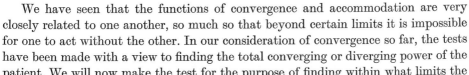

We have seen that the functions of convergence and accommodation are very closely related to one another, so much so that beyond certain limits it is impossible for one to act without the other. In our consideration of convergence so far, the tests have been made with a view to finding the total converging or diverging power of the patient. We will now make the test for the purpose of finding within what limits the convergence may act without influencing the accommodation. That is, to what extent the convergence may exert or relax its power while the accommodation is fixed for any given point. How may this be done? Moving any object closer or farther from the eye would not answer our purpose, for at every change of position the accommodation and convergence would act in harmony with one another which is precisely as Nature intends. We can however, place an object at a certain distance from the eye, and by placing prisms before the eyes, induce the convergence to act without changing the accommodation. For instance if we place an object one meter in front of the eyes, there will be one meter-angle of convergence used and (the patient being an emmetrope) one dioptre of accommodation. If now we place prisms before the eyes, bases out, the convergence will be increased, but as prisms do not change the relative direction of rays, (that is, leaving them the same divergence as before, the whole pencil of rays being bent alike) the accommodation will remain the same. By continuing to increase the prismatic power we are enabled to find the strongest prism through which he can still see the object distinctly and singly. We now take the prisms off and still directing the patient to look toward the object, place the prisms before him bases in. He is now using less than one meter-angle of convergence but is still using a dioptre of accommodation. As we continue to increase the prisms the convergence must necessarily relax until we reach the limit when the accommodation must also relax, thus giving indistinct vision, or else the convergence will refuse to act further, thus creating diplopia. The strongest prism base in which he can overcome, is the limit of his power to relax convergence while the accommodation is fixed.

The difference between the two points, that is the range covered by the convergence in changing from the point of greatest relaxation to the point of greatest exertion, while the accommodation remains fixed for a certain point is called "Relative Convergence." Copy:

> *83. Relative Convergence is the total amount of converging power which the eyes are capable of exerting, independently of accommodation. That is, it is the limit, both of exertion and relaxation of convergence, the accommodation remaining fixed for one point.*

If we desire to find the limit of accommodation, the convergence remaining fixed, we will use spherical lenses instead of prisms. Requesting the patient to fix his gaze upon some object, at whatever distance we may desire to make the test, we first place convex lenses before his eyes. These lenses will have no effect upon the convergence but will increase the refraction of the eye, thereby causing the accommodation to relax in order to still hold the image upon the retina. If we continue to add convex lenses until it is impossible for the accommodation to relax farther unless the convergence can also relax, we have reached the limit, and the vision will be imperfect, or diplopia will be produced. The strongest convex glass then through which he can still see distinctly will measure the limit in that direction. We now remove the glasses and place concave lenses before his eyes. The convergence still remains undisturbed, but the refraction of the eye is decreased by the minus lenses, thus calling upon the accommodation to make an effort in order to replace the deficiency. With every addition of the minus power the accommodation is increased until the limit is reached, when vision again becomes either indistinct or double. The strongest concave glass which can be overcome of course measures the limit in this direction.

Let us suppose that our patient is an emmetrope and that we direct him to look at an object 50 cm away. He will of course use 2 D of accommodation and 2 M. A. of convergence. We now place a convex glass of 1 D before each eye, he says he still sees the object as distinctly as before. Next we place a plus 0.50 D in front of the 1 D making a total of 1.50 D. With this he says that he sees two of the objects instead of one. We know then that the 1.50 D was too strong so we decide to try 1.25 D. This can be done by taking off the 0.50 D and replacing it with a 0.25 D; or we can take both lenses off and replace them with a 1.25 D; or we can get the same result by leaving both the 1.00 D and 0.50 D before the eyes, and placing in front of them a minus 0.25. At any rate we try the plus 1.25 D and find that he again sees distinctly and singly. This tells us that he is capable of relaxing his accommodation just 1.25 D and no more, while the convergence remains fixed. After removing the convex lenses we try concaves in the same manner and we find that the strongest he can overcome is 1 D. We now know that he is capable of exercising his accommodation over a range of 2.25 D independently of his converging power. This 2.25 D is called his "Relative Accommodation." Copy:

84. Relative Accommodation is the total amount of accommodative power which the eyes are capable of exercising, independently of convergence.

Do not confuse relative accommodation and convergence with the total amount of these powers. For instance, in our last examples the patient could have easily accommodated a number of dioptres more had the convergence also been allowed to act. The term "relative" is applied only to the amount of power one of these functions is capable of exerting while the other is stationary.

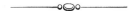

Accommodation and convergence being so intimately linked together we can readily understand that should these functions be disturbed beyond their relative limits, serious conditions and anomalies may arise. So far we have always considered the patients under tests to be emmetropes, in which case the two functions work harmoniously together, every dioptre of accommodation being accompanied by a corresponding meter-angle of convergence. If the patient is a myope of hypermetrope the conditions will be different. Let us first consider the hypermetropic eye. This eye being shorter than its focal length, the principal focus will fall behind the retina, and he must, even when looking at distant objects, exert his accommodation in order to bring the image forward. At the same time however the convergence must not act, for the object is at infinity, hence the rays are coming parallel. If for example our patient is a hypermetrope of 1 D he must use 1 D of accommodation at all times in order to see distinctly at infinity, but of course uses no convergence. If he looks at an object one meter away he uses 2 D of accommodation but only 1 M. A. of convergence; if one-half meter away he uses 3 D of accommodation and 2 M. A. of convergence, always holding back his convergence one meter-angle less than the accommodation. A hypermetrope of 2 D must always use 2 D more accommodation than he uses meter-angles of convergence; a hypermetrope of 4 D uses 4 D more and so on. We have learned that there is a limit to the distance which accommodation and convergence may work apart from one another, and that after the limit is reached both must act together.

Let us suppose that we have a patient whose eyes are 10 D hypermetropic. In order for this person to bring parallel rays to a focus upon his retina he must use 10 D of accommodation, but must use no convergence as his eyes must be held parallel to receive these rays. Now it is impossible for the accommodation to exert itself that amount independently of convergence, as 10 D is certainly beyond the limit of relative accommodation. He can do one of two things as he chooses. Either give up trying to accommodate at all and be satisfied with a blurred, indistinct image, thus making his vision equally as poor as that of a myope of the same degree, or he may accommodate the 10 D but must of course allow his convergence to act at the same time. In the latter case the result is simply cross-eye, nothing more or less.

The question naturally arises: Why does not a cross-eyed person see double? If both eyes are good this is usually the case for the first few months after the habit has begun to form, and the eyes will oscillate backward and forward seeming to hesitate between the two alternatives of seeing double or relaxing the accommodation. I have had children come to me in this condition, whose parents say that they always cover one eye with their hand when reading, or using their eyes in any unusual way. This is easy to understand, for by covering the one eye it can turn as far as it pleases without producing diplopia. After a little however the patient learns to suppress the sensation received upon one retina, and is soon able to keep both eyes open without noticing the image formed in the squinting eye at all. A watchmaker in using his eye glass keeps both eyes open but only sees with one eye, paying no attention to the other, so that sometimes another person may enter the room and pass his hand in front of that eye without the watchmaker being conscious of his presence. If one eye of the child is naturally a poor eye, having imperfect vision to begin with, it becomes much easier for the habit to form, as there is not much inducement for the poor eye to remain straight. The majority of cross-eyed people are found with the crossed eye very inferior to the other, although there are a few exceptions. The rule however, is, that in those cases of high hypermetropia where vision is equally good in each eye, the desire for single vision is much stronger than the desire for distinct vision, and the patient chooses the alternative of not accommodating, and thus escapes strabismus at the sacrifice of clear images. You can certainly see what a blessing convex lenses must be to those hypermetropic persons, for not only is the excessive work of the accommodation relieved, but at the same stroke convergence and accommodation are brought into working harmony, and if the strabismus is not of too long standing, it will be soon overcome.

In myopia the result is just the opposite of hypermetropia. In looking at an infinite distance the convergence and accommodation are of course at rest, the eye having to be content with blurred images, as there is no way by which the focus can be thrown back to the retina except with concave lenses. We therefore have no strain when looking at infinity, but when the object is brought nearer the convergence must at once begin to act, while the accommodation remains passive waiting for the focus to reach the retina. If the myopia is of 2 D, the object must be brought to one-half meter before the eyes in order to give distinct vision. The convergence then makes an exertion of 2 M. A. with the accommodation at rest. This of course is contrary to the natural tendency and explains why near-sighted people complain of their eyes tiring when reading. If we consider only the refractive condition of the eye we would naturally suppose that reading would be very easy for the myope, since he is already adapted for a near point and of course would not have to use his accommodation. This would be true had the myope but one eye, but the accommodation and convergence are so intimately linked that it would produce much less strain if the myope could be allowed to use his accommodation in harmony with his convergence, than to be compelled to hold it back.

Theoretically there would be two ways of overcoming this disturbance, one by concave lenses, thus allowing his accommodation to act, the other by prisms base in; which will let him look at a near object without converging. The latter would not be practical however, for as soon as he looks toward infinity he must remove the prisms, else his eyes will be diverging while accommodation is still at rest. Besides his vision would still be imperfect for distance, so that the prisms would be of no use to him except as a temporary means of relief when reading, while with concave lenses we not only place the two functions in working harmony, but at the same time give the patient distinct vision for all distances, in fact make him an emmetrope, which is always our aim in fitting glasses.

In high degree of myopia where the limits of relative convergence and accommodation are over-reached, the eyes remain perfectly at rest when looking at a distance, but when the object is close, convergence is expected to act without accommodation. As it is impossible for the two to remain so far apart he must either accommodate also, and be satisfied with indistinct vision for near as well as for distance, or he must refuse to converge, thus leaving his eyes parallel while looking at close objects. In the latter case he of course sees the object with but one eye, the other turning outward. This habit gradually forming, the eyes will eventually remain divergent at all times, creating what is known as "Divergent Strabismus," the opposite of cross-eye. Concave lenses used in time would have prevented this condition by placing the two functions in working harmony with one another.

For your study between mails read the entire third chapter of Hartridge.

(End of Lesson No. 8.)

QUESTIONS ON LESSON NO. 8.

138. What is Convergence?

139. How do you measure convergence?

140. How do you find the punctum remotum of convergence?

141. How much convergence will a person use in looking at an object 30 feet away?

142. 30 inches away?

143. What relation exists between accommodation and convergence? Explain fully.

144. Give your understanding of relative convergence.

145. Of relative accommodation.

146. How much accommodation and how much convergence will be used by a hypermetrope of 2 D in looking at an object 6 meters away?

147. In looking at an object 20 cm away?

148. How much of each will be used by a myope of 3 D in looking toward an object 30 feet away?

149. In looking at an object 8 cm away?

150. Explain what defects of the eye will cause converging and diverging strabismus and why, and in what way each may be prevented.

EXPLANATIONS ON LESSONS NO. 7 AND NO. 8.

111. Accommodation is the inherent power of the eye to change its adjustment so as to clearly focus rays coming from objects at different distances.

112. The action of the Cilliary Muscle upon the Suspensory Ligaments which hold the crystalline lens in place loosens their tension upon the lens and allows it from its own elasticity to become more convex. When the Cilliary Muscles relax, the ligaments again resume their tension and the lens is again brought to a state of least convexity. The action of the cilliary muscle therefore causes the lens to assume any desired power (within certain limits) and in that way adjusts the eye for the desired distance.

113. The power of accommodation gradually decreases from the age of ten until at seventy-five it is entirely gone.

114. The Punctum Proximum (Latin for near point).   115. The accommodative power is exerted to the utmost.

116. The Punctum Remotum (Latin for far point). The accommodation is at rest. 117. The Range is the DISTANCE between the far and near points. The Amplitude is the POWER used in changing from the far to the near point.

118. In emmetropia, at infinity; in myopia, at a finite distance; in hypermetropia, a negative point behind the eye.

119. If the P. R. is behind the eye he is a hypermetrope. The distance, 10 cm. tells us that he is a hypermetrope of 10 D. (100 divided by 10 equals 10). In other words his lens is 10 D. too weak for the length of his eye. (See answer to No. 103). He must therefore accommodate 10 D in order to make his lens equal in strength to that of an emmetrope. Therefore in accommodating 14D he has used 10 D to make himself emmetropic and the other 4 D to adjust for a near point. In other words this hypermetrope of 10 D when accommodating 14 D is equal to an emmetrope accommodating 4 D. His near point (punctum proximum) is at 25 cm.

120. An emmetrope would use 5 D of accommodation to see at 20 cm. This eye sees there with only 3 D. Hence his lens must be naturally 2 D stronger than that of an emmetrope which proves him to be a myope 2 D. Therefore his P. R. is 50 cm in front of the eye.

121. An emmetrope uses 5 D to see at 20 cm. This eye can only reach that point with 8D. He must therefore have used the extra 3 D to bring his focus to the retina. Hence he is a 3 D and his P. R. is 33 1/3 cm behind the eye.

122. As he has used just the right amount of accommodation to see at his near point, his eye must be just right, or emmetropic.

123. At infinity. (*Rule 79.*)

124. An emmetrope uses 1 D of accommodation to adjust for 1 M. However this patient is not an emmetrope but a myope of one-half D for he can only see 2 M away. Therefore his lens is already one-half D stronger than that of an emmetrope so, in looking a 1 M he will use one-half D less than the emmetrope. Answer: 0.50 D.

125. The P. R. tells us that the eye is hypermetropic 2 D. In order for him to see objects, even at infinity, he will have to use 2 D of accommodation to bring the focus to his retina. As he has but 1 D of accommodative power, he cannot do this, but can only bring his focus half way to the retina, thus overcoming but half of his defect. This will leave him a hypermetrope of 1 D. He is when at rest, a hypermetrope of 2 D and when at work a hypertrope of 1 D. His P. R. therefore is at 50 cm negative and the P. P. at 1 M negative. 1 M behind the eye is the correct answer.

126. An emmetrope uses 12.50 D of accommodation to adjust for 8 cm. A myope of 2 D

has a lens that is already 2 D stronger than the emmetrope's. Therefore he will have 2 D less work to do in adjusting for the same point. Answer: 10.50 D.

127. The range is the distance between the far and the near point. The far point of a 3 D myope is 33 1/3 cm in front of him. If his lens is already 3 D too strong and he has the power to increase it 3 D more, he swells it up until it is 6 D too strong and makes himself temporarily a 6 D myope. Hence his near point is 16 2/3 cm in front of him. If his P. P. is 16 2/3 cm away and his P R 33 1/3 cm away, his range is the distance between the two which is 16 2/3 cm.

128. The P. R. of a 5 D myope is at 20 cm. If he can increase his lens 3 D more he makes himself a myope of 8 D and his P. P. is therefore at 12 1/2 cm. Hence his range is the distance between the two which is 7 1/2 cm.

129. Compare this with No. 119 and you will find it is the same patient. He is a hypermetrope of 10 D.   130. 10 cm behind the eye.

131. The far point, or resting place, of a 0.50 D myope is at 2 M. As he is 80 years of age he has no power to change his adjustment and therefore 2 M is his far point, near point and only point. Answer: 2 meters.

132. An emmetrope uses 4 D to see 25 cm. This eye used 3 D more to see at the same point. Hence it is hypermetropic 3 D and the correcting glass is plus 3 D.

133. An ammetrope uses 10 D to see at 10 cm. This eye reached the same point with 3 D less. Hence it is myopic 3 D and the correcting glass is minus 3 D.

134. An emmetrope uses 8 D to see at 12 1/2 cm. This eye has used the same. Hence it is emmetropic and needs no correcting glass.

135. 3 M represents an accommodative effort of one-third D. 2 M. represents an effort of 1/2 D. The amount of accommodation necessary to change from one point to the other would therefore be the difference between 1/3 D and 1/2 which is 1/6. Written 0.16 D.

136. 1 M represents an effort of 1 D. One-half meter (or 50 cm) represents an effort of 2 D. The accommodation necessary to change from one point to the other is the difference between 1 D and 2 D which is 1 D.

137. I hope that every one of you have done so for I have arranged the rules so as to make you a complete reference book that will be of value to you every day you are in practice.

I realize that Lesson No. 7 has been difficult for most of you, but if you will study carefully the supplement and the explanations I believe you will be able to master it. Give it especial study as all of the succeeding lessons hinge upon a thorough understanding of these subjects.

138. The act of turning the two eyes in toward a near object.

139. By a system similar to the dioptric system, except that we use the term "Meter-Angle" instead of "dioptre."

140. By having the patient look at a flame 6 meters or more away and placing prisms before the eyes, bases in, as long as single vision is maintained. This gives us the amount of diverging power, or negative convergence. The P. R. is behind the eye.

141. As 30 feet is an infinite distance, rays will come parallel and no convergence is necessary.

142. To reduce from the inch to the dioptric system divide 40 inches by the given number. 40 divided by 30 gives us one and one-third M. A.

143. In every pair of eyes whether emmetropic, myopic or hypermetropic, if the accommodation acts a certain number of dioptres the convergence WANTS to act the same number of meter-angles and is uncomfortable if not allowed to do so. Beyond certain limits it is bound to do so regardless of the will power.

144. The amount that the eyes can converge and still hold the accommodation fixed.

145. The amount the eyes can accommodate and still hold the convergence fixed.

146. 2 D of accommodation to make up his weak lens. No convergence as the rays come parallel.

147. 7 D of accommodation and 5 M A of convergence.

148. No accommodation for it would make him more myopic than ever. No convergence for the rays come parallel. He will however see indistinctly at that distance.

149. 9.50 D of accommodation and 12.50 M A of convergence.

150. Converging Strabismus is caused by a high degree of hypermetropia because when the accommodation acts to bring the focus to the retina the convergence is bound to turn the eyes in (answer 143.) Convex lenses remove the cause for accommodating and as the accommodation goes to rest convergence also goes to rest and the eyes are straight. I hope no student of mine will ever be guilty of using prisms in cross eye nor of recommending an operation until it has been proved beyond a doubt that plus lenses will not correct the defect. Diverging Strabismus is caused by myopia of high degree, because in bringing objects near either the accommodation must act or the convergence go to rest. In the latter case the eyes form the habit of remaining too far apart and diverging strabismus finally results. Concave lenses would have prevented it.

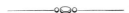

I have received quite a number of letters this week asking if we could still supply the set of 20 lessons in book form instead of the loose leaves. We only had enough made up to fill the orders that came in at the beginning of the course, but as so many have expressed a desire for them we have decided to make up another edition. This edition will, as before, be just sufficient to fill the actual number of cash orders received, as we do not wish to have any left over. The price will still be one dollar, but in addition I would ask that you kindly return the lessons and questions already sent as each belongs to a set. The book form is an advantage not only during the course but as a reference book afterward, and is really worth much more than the dollar difference. As this is the last edition we will have made up kindly send your order at once so that we may arrange accordingly.

Thanking you all for the interest you are taking in the work I remain with kindest regards,

Yours Sincerely,

Dr. H. A. Thomson.

LESSON NO. 9.

Subjective Examinations.

IF WE COULD know at once just the refractive condition of every eye that comes to us, it would be a very simple matter to prescribe the correcting glass in each instance. If it is myopic 2 D we would give a minus glass of that strength, if hypermetropic, a plus glass. But how to determine these conditions and the exact amount of defect is the question which now confronts us. We cannot open the eye and examine its lens and retina, nor can we remove it from the orbit to measure its length. We must therefore devise some other method of determining the refraction without resorting to such extreme measures. A great many ingenious methods have been suggested, all of which are more or less valuable, and it is always advisable to make use of two or more of them when making an examination, in order to prove the accuracy of our work.

The study and consideration of the different methods of examination, is called "Dioptometry" meaning "the measure of the eye." It is divided into two general classes "Subjective" and "Objective." Copy:

85. *Subjective Examinations are those in which rays entering the eye are considered. That is, we consider the sensations produced upon the patient's retina, basing our judgment upon his answers.*

86. *Objective Examinations are those in which rays emerging from the eye are considered. That is, we consider the images formed by rays leaving the retina, and draw our conclusions without questioning the patient.*

This lesson will consider some of the subjective methods of examination, viz.: The Acuteness of Vision, the chromatic Test, Optometry, etc. The method based upon acuteness of vision is the most important and accurate test we have, and is conducted by means of the trial case and test types. The test types consist of letters of graduated sizes, constructed upon accurate measurement. The nerve ends of the retina are made up of alternating rods and cones distributed in regular order along the surface of the retina, being closer together at the macula than at the periphery. It has been found that in order for the eye to distinguish form or outline, enough rays must touch the retina to disturb at least two cones at a time. Any amount less than this will only disturb one rod and one cone, thereby only creating a sensation of light but no distinction of form. The visual angle formed by rays from the extreme points of any object must be at least an angle of one minute in size in order to obtain this result. Test types are therefore constructed on this principle.

Each letter is made of just such a size that when it is placed at the distance intended, the rays from it will form a one minute angle in the eye. For instance, we wish to make a certain letter to be seen at a distance of 200 feet. Measurements are taken and it is found that an object 200 feet away must be of a certain size in order to form a one minute angle in the eye. Accordingly each arm of the letter is made of that size, the whole letter being large enough to form a five minute angle. Now an eye which can read this letter at 200 feet has average acuteness of vision and we call his vision 200/200 of 1. Letters to be seen at nearer points are also made, one for 70 feet, one for 40 feet, 30 feet, 20 feet, etc. Each letter, or row of letters is numbered, either in meters or feet, or sometimes both, and we have what is known as Snellen's Test Types. If an eye is not able to read the 200 foot letter at 200 feet, the visual acuteness is not average but is below the standard. If it is necessary to bring the card up to 80 feet before he is able to name the letter, his vision is only 80/200 as good as the standard vision, and we say his vision equals 80/200. By this method we have a simple and accurate means of expressing the visual acuteness, always taking the distance at which the patient reads for numerator, and the distance at which the letter should be read, as the denominator of our fraction. Copy:

> 87. *The visual acuteness of an eye is expressed by a fraction, the numerator being the distance at which the letter is read, and the denominator the distance at which it should be read.*

Where will we hang our test types? If less than 20 feet away the accommodation will be called upon to act and we are thus prevented from getting the measure of the eye at rest. More than 20 feet will be perfectly correct, but few rooms are built longer than 20 feet and as that distance answers every purpose it has become customary to hang the cards just that distance (6 meters) away. We now seat our patient and ask him to read aloud the smallest line of type which he can make out. If he reads the 6 meter line we say that his vision is average and record it V equals 6/6, or if we are considering feet, 20/20. It is however, becoming more customary with the profession every day to use the metric system exclusively and we will therefore confine our computations hereafter to that system of measurement. We say then that V equals 6/6. If he only reads the 10 M line we say V equals 6/10, etc.

Let us suppose that our patient's vision for the right eye (the left eye being covered with a disc) equals 6/6. We know at once that he is not a myope, for a myope could not see so distinctly as to meters. He may be a hypermetrope, for a hypermetrope has only to use sufficient accommodation to bring the focus forward upon the retina, thus making his vision as good as the emmetropes; or he may be an emmetrope. How are we to determine between these two conditions? Let us consider them. If he is a hypermetrope he must certainly be using some accommodation; if an emmetrope he is using none. If we place a plus glass before a hypermetropic eye will he see better or worse? Before giving him the glass his accommodation was in use holding the image upon the retina, but when the plus glass is added it takes the place of his accommodation, and, he relaxes the effort. The image is however, still upon the retina and he reads exactly the same line as before, seeing neither better nor worse, but just the same. Placing the plus glass before him does not effect the image in the least but simply relaxes the accommodation. If we alternately remove and replace the glass a number of times the crystalline lens will increase and decrease in convexity accordingly, the image always remaining upon the retina and the vision always remaining the same. If we place a plus glass before an emmetropic eye the result will be different. His accommodation is already at rest so that he cannot relax, and the glass adding to the refraction of his eye will bring rays to a focus before reaching the retina thus making him artificially myopic. Vision will of course be worse.

We have then a very simple and effective means of determining the condition. Asking our patient to again look toward the test types, we place a weak plus glass before his eye, for instance an 0.50 D, and ask him if he can see just as well. If he says he cannot we remove it and try a 0.25 D. If he still says that he cannot see as well as without it we know that he is an emmetrope. If on the other hand, he says that the 0.50 D is just as good as without, we know he is a hypermetrope of at least that amount, so we proceed to try a stronger lens, say a 0.75 D. If he still continues to read the 6/6 line we keep on increasing the strength until he says he cannot see as well. We know then that his accommodation has relaxed all it will, and that now the image is lifted off the retina making him myopic. The strongest plus glass with which he still sees as well as without, is the measure of his hypermetropia. Copy:

88. The strongest convex glass through which an eye can still maintain its best vision is the measure of the manifest hypermetropia.

We now uncover the left eye, placing the disc before the right, and again proceed in the same manner taking the strongest plus glass which he will accept as the measure of his hypermetropia. One point more and the test is finished. The hypermetropic eye, from its long habit of accommodating for all distances is sometimes very slow to relax all of its accommodation. We therefore find it necessary after fitting both eyes separately, to remove the disc and with both uncovered try to induce them to accept a little stronger glass. To do this we will take a 0.25 D in each hand, holding one before either eye, and again ask him if he sees as well. If he does, we continue to increase the strength until the limit is again reached, stopping at the strongest glass with which he still maintains distinct vision. We are often enabled to induce the accommodation to relax to a considerable extent in this way after the eyes had refused any stronger lens while tested separately. Sometimes it is impossible with all our efforts to induce the accommodation to entirely relax, the old habit being so firmly fixed, and in that case there remains a portion of the hypermetropia which we cannot bring out by the use of this test. That portion is called "Latent Hypermetropia," as a distinction between it and that which is easily brought out, which we call the "Manifest Hypermetropia." For the present however we will only consider the manifest, as the majority of our patients will readily relax the accommodation making it an easy matter to determine the exact amount of the defect. Latent Hypermetropia will be considered later, in the lesson on spasm of the accommodation.

If instead of reading 6/6 our patient can only read the 6/12 line, myopia is to be suspected. Still we cannot say positively that it is myopia, as there are many causes for low visual acuteness. The retina may be impaired, the optic nerve diseased, or perhaps lens cornea, or one of the humors is cloudy or opaque. Astigmatism, which we will consider later, may be present, or the eye may be hypermetropic and lack sufficient accommodative power to bring the focus upon the retina. If owing to some disease, the case is not for us as opticians, but should be referred to an oculist or physician, but if the poor vision is owing to defective refraction, as Myopia, Hypermetropia, Astigmatism, etc., it is our business to correct the defect and thus give the eye clear, distinct images upon the retina. It is necessary therefore, that we determine once and for all to which class of troubles the defective vision may be attributed, and we have a very simple and easy method of deciding this question, viz.: the pin-hole test.

The pin-hole test consists of an opaque disc, set in a metal rim the same as the trial lens, having at its center a small aperture not larger than a pin. This we place in the trial frame and set before the patient's eye, asking him at the same time if he can read any more letters when looking through it. If he can the case is one of refractive error, and can be corrected by glasses. If not, the poor vision is owing to some imperfect condition of the eye's tissues, and should be referred to an oculist. How can such a simple contrivance decide so important a question? This can be easily understood if we consider the nature of the two conditions. In the case of diseased or imperfect tissues, a perfect image may be thrown upon the retina, in fact the eye may be perfectly emmetropic, but if the retina or nerves fail to respond readily to the impression the acuteness of vision will of course be low. In the case of refractive error the vision is poor because the rays entering the eye are not focussed to a point, but fall upon the retina in circles of diffusion, as shown in diagram A. Let L represent the crystalline lens, H a hypermetropic retina, and M a myopic one. Upon each of these retinae a diffusion circle "ab" is formed, instead of a distinct point as would be the case were the retina

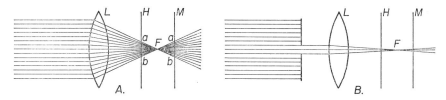

placed at F. Vision is therefore imperfect. Let us now place the pin-hole disc before the eye as in Diagram B. All of the outer rays are now cut off, only those being admitted which are upon, or near to the principal axis. These rays strike the retina close together and form a very distinct point. It is evident then, that if the pin-hole test improves vision, a lens whose business it is to bring all rays to a focus upon the retina would improve it still more, but if the low vision is owing to disease of the eye tissues or nerves, it need not be attributed to blurred images.

Let us suppose that our patient reads 6/12 and that by placing the pin-hole before him he can read a line better. We know that a refractive error exists so we may proceed with the examination. Although we suspect myopia it is always best to try the plus lenses first, for it may be some other defect, and plus lenses always have a tendency toward relaxing the accommodation, while minus lenses, when placed before an eye which does not require them, always have an influence in setting the accommodation at work, which we wish to avoid. We remove the pin-hole disc then, and try a weak plus lens, but in this case the patient says he sees worse. We therefore remove the plus and try a minus. With this he can see better. We now know that it is a case of myopia and that the lens has moved the focus back nearer to the retina thus making him see more distinctly. We try a little stronger lens and he sees still better. We continue to add minus lenses until they no longer improve vision stopping at the weakest one through which he still sees as well. Let us suppose that the first lens given him was a minus 0.50 D with which he could see considerably better. The next (minus 1.00 D) improves the vision and we try a 1.25 D. He says that this is just as good as the 1.00 D, in fact, he can see no difference in them. What will we do in this case? If the 1.25 D gives just the same vision as the 1.00 D it is certainly no improvement, hence the image is no nearer the retina than it was before. Every minus lens carries the focus backward, and the fact that he sees equally as well with one as the other must indicate that the accommodation has been taking a part in the work and that the focus was upon the retina both times, for he is certainly seeing at his best. The 1.00 D is the measure of his myopia then, for we can readily see that the 1.25 D simply threw the focus back of the retina and the accommodation brought it forward again. We might continue to add minus lenses so long as the accommodative strength is able to overcome them, but what a punishment it would be to the patient. It is our business to relieve him of all surplus work and strain and we surely cannot do so by giving the accommodation work to do. Every minus glass we add after the focus has touched the retina simply makes the eye that much hypermetropic and as our aim is to make eyes emmetropic this would hardly be consistent. The weaker glass then is the correction. Copy:

89. *The weakest concave glass through which an eye can obtain its best vision is the measure of the myopia.*

In making these tests be careful not to confuse the acuteness of vision with the refraction. A great many pupils form the idea that 6/6 represents the emmetropic eye and that the hypermetropic and myopic eyes have certain other lines representing them, and that if an eye does not read 6/6 it is not an emmetrope. This is not the idea I would have you form. The visual acuteness simply expresses how well the eye can see, the average being 6/6 for an eye whose focus is upon the retina. An eye may however be perfectly emmetropic and still only read 6/10 or 6/12 owing to the retina not having so great sensibility; or on the other hand a hypermetrope may read 6/4 with the aid of his accommodation, on account of good retinal perception. We always aim to raise the visual acuteness as high as possible but of course can go no farther than to bring a clear image upon the retina. We make a record of the vision both with and without glasses so that a glance shows us just what improvement the lenses have given.

The different lenses in all the numbers, both concave and convex, together with the trial frames, pin-hole tests and all the other necessary appurtenances are furnished with every good trial case. This constitutes the most important and accurate method of fitting glasses that we have, although many of the other tests are very valuable.

Chromatic Test.

This test is based upon the principles of chromatic aberration. One eye being covered we place before the other a plane, cobalt-blue glass. This glass is capable of transmitting only the red and blue rays, all others being absorbed. We direct the patient to look at a candle or gas flame 6 meters away. The light after passing through the

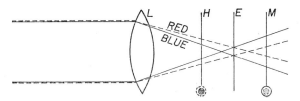

glass is deprived of all rays save the red and blue, and these approach the eye together forming a red-blue (cobalt-blue) light. Upon entering the eye these rays are refracted by the cornea and lens toward the macula, but, as we learned in Lesson No. 5, the blue rays are refracted more than the red, and will therefore come to a focus first. In the diagram, L represents the crystalline lens, H a hypermetropic, E an emmetropic, and M a myopic retina. The hypermetrope H, catches the rays before they come to a focus, the blue being on the inside, the red outside. He sees the flame of a blue color with a red margin or halo. The emmetrope E catches the rays as they are about to cross one another and therefore sees the flame as a cobalt blue. The rays having crossed before reaching the myope M, the red is now on the inside and the blue without. He will of course see a red flame with a blue halo. This is a most excellent preliminary test as it shows us at once what class of defect we have to deal with, the only objection being that in young hypermetropes the accommodation overcomes the hypermetropia and they of course see the same as emmetropes. It never fails us though in myopia (unless the patient is color-blind, which is due to an absence or undevelopment of some of the nerve fibers of the retina) as the accommodation is powerless to overcome myopia, and in older patients it is equally as efficient in determining hypermetropia. To find the amount of defect we can place plus or minus lenses before the eyes until the light is of a cobalt blue, when we know we have made him emmetropic. In hypermetropia the strongest plus glass with which he still sees the light cobalt-blue would be the measure of his defect, for as soon as the glass is too strong he would see the light as a myope. The chromatic test is not of course perfectly accurate owing to the patients' inability to determine just when he sees the light at its best, but as a preliminary test, giving us the defect and an approximate idea of its degree, the test is certainly a valuable one.

Optometry.

Although I hope none of my pupils will ever be so unscientific as to use an optometer, it is desirable to understand the principles upon which it is constructed. The common optometer consists of a convex lens through which the patient looks at a card attached to a slide. The card is moved until seen most distinctly, when we have the focus of that eye. If it stopped at the principal focus of the lens we know that the rays emerged parallel and that he is emmetropic. If beyond the principal focus they emerged converging showing him to be hypermetropic; if nearer than the focus, diverging, and he is myopic. By marking the slide at different distances we have only to look where the card stands and the number tells the glass required. Other more complicated optometers are upon the market, but are based upon the same principle. The objection is that accommodation, convergence, astigmatism, etc., are not considered, thus rendering the instruments inaccurate.

Between mails study Hartridge Chapters 4 and 5 omitting the parts relating to Astigmatism.

QUESTIONS ON LESSON NO. 9.

151. What is meant by Subjective Examination?

152. Objective Examination?

153. What is the rule in correcting hypermetropia?

154. In correcting myopia?

155. What do we mean when we say that the visual acuteness of an eye is 6/12?

156. When we say it is 6/6?

157. If the visual acuteness if 6/18 how do we determine whether the trouble is due to Ametropia or to disease? Explain the principle of the test?

158. How will you proceed in making a test for myopia?

159. Explain the test for Hypermetropia?

160. Give your understanding of the chromatic test.

LESSON NO. 10.

Objective Examinations.

WE WILL NOW consider the rays of light as they proceed FROM the eye of the patient, forming our judgment of the defect by the direction which the rays take. The retina of the emmetropic eye is situated at the principal focus of the dioptric system, hence parallel rays entering the eye come to a focus upon it. If on the other hand we consider the retina as the object, light will leave the eye in parallel rays. In the myopic eye the retina is beyond the principal focus and it is necessary that we bring an object to some finite distance, thus giving the eye diverging rays, in order to bring the conjugate upon the retina. If the retina is taken as the object, the rays will emerge converging toward the punctum remotum. The hypermetropic eye requires converging rays to focus on the retina, hence if we take the retina for our object (it being in front of the principal focus) the rays will leave diverging. We can then deduct the following rules. Copy: "*OBJECTIVE EXAMINATIONS.*"

90. Rays leaving the retina of an emmetropic eye will emerge parallel.

91. Rays leaving the retina of a myopic eye will emerge converging.

92. Rays leaving the retina of a hypermetropic eye will emerge diverging.

Among the most important objective tests are those made with the Ophthalmoscope. This instrument consists of a concave mirror having a small sight-hole through its center, and is mounted upon a handle. Behind the mirror is a circular disc, made to revolve upon its center, in which is set lenses of different powers. By turning this disc any lens we desire to use may be thrown in front of the sight-hole, the lenses being numbered so that we may tell at a glance just what lens is before us.

In order for light to come to us from the retina, the retina must be illuminated, for we know that the interior of the eye is kept dark by the iris. It is for the purpose of lighting up the eye that the concave mirror is used. Seating the patient in the chair we place a lamp or gas burner behind him, either over his head or to one side. We now hold the ophthalmoscope before him in such a position that the light from the lamp will be reflected by the mirror straight into his eye, thus lighting up the interior. If now, we look through the peep-hole in the center of the mirror we will be directly in line with the reflected light and will be able to distinctly see the retina, together with arteries and veins of the chlorid, provided we have our eye in focus for that point. We will now consider the methods of determining the refraction of the eye by the use of this instrument. The art of using the ophthalmoscope is called "Ophthalmoscopy," pronounced with the accent on the syllable "mos." Copy:

93. The study of the ophthalmoscope is called "Ophthalmoscopy."

94. Ophthalmoscopy is divided into three methods of examination. The Direct
   Method; the Indirect Method; and the Concave Mirror at a Distance.

The Direct Method.

Let us suppose that the patient and yourself are both emmetropic, and that neither of you have any accommodation. The only rays which you can focus upon your retina are parallel rays. Light coming from the patient's retina will of course be parallel, so you have only to look through the empty sight-hole of the ophthalmoscope in order to see his retina very distinctly. Hartridge Fig. 46 shows the course of the rays in such a case. If your patient is a hypermetrope the rays will leave his eye diverging, and if your eye is still emmetropic with no accommodation, you will be unable to see his retina distinctly as the focus for these diverging rays will fall behind your retina. In order to obtain a good view, it will be necessary to place a plus lens before your eye of sufficient power to bring the focus to your retina, or in other words to make the diverging rays from his eye come to your eye parallel. This you do by turning up the plus lenses of the ophthalmoscope. Hartridge Fig. 47 shows the course of the rays in such an instance. E representing your emmetropic eye, and H the hypermetropic eye of the patient. Rays leaving the eye take the direction of the diverging dotted lines, but are intercepted by the plus glass and so bent that they enter your eye parallel which is what you require. If now with the convex glass before his eye, rays leaving his retina emerge from the glass parallel, it must be clear by Rule 29 that rays of light coming from infinity and passing through this glass will come to a focus upon his retina. The lens therefore having made him emmetropic must be his correcting glass, and you have only to look at the number of the lens to determine the degree of his hypermetropia.

If your patient is a myope the rays will leave his eye converging, and as your eye is still adapted for parallel rays, you will not see the retina distinctly. In order to make these rays parallel so that you can focus them upon your retina, we must place a concave glass between your eye and his. This you can do by turning up the lenses in the ophthalmoscope. Hartridge Fig. 48 shows such a case. If rays leaving the retina will emerge from this glass parallel, it must according to Rule 29, be the correcting glass for his eye, the number of the lens showing the degree of his myopia.

In making this test I have considered your eye to be emmetropic and without accommodation. How can this be brought about? Every optician is certainly not emmetropic and there are but few who do not possess a considerable amount of accommodation. The refractive errors may be overcome by the optician putting on his correcting glasses before making the test. He will then of course be emmetropic. If he has no glasses he can deduct the amount of his defect from the lens used in the ophthalmoscope. For instance if he is a hypermetrope of 1 D, and the lens used in the ophthalmoscope, to give a distinct view of the retina, is convex 3 D we know the patient to be a hypermetrope of 2 D. If the lens used is a concave 3 D we know him to be a myope of 4 D. If the optician is a myope he must make allowance for his defect in just the opposite way, adding to the plus lens and subtracting from the minus lens.

To dispose of the accommodation is much more difficult. The optician must learn to hold his cilliary muscle as much under control as he does other muscles of his body. This requires long and constant practice but can be attained very perfectly after a few months experience. This is the only objection to the direct method as it is difficult for the beginner to relax his accommodation and to hold it in a relaxed condition during the entire test. To practice this the pupil can begin by looking through a window screen at some object across the street, and without changing the direction of his eyes look at the screen itself, alternating this movement a few times until he feels conscious of a movement going on in his eyes, always stopping before the exercise becomes tiresome. By doing this several times a day he soon begins to recognize the action of the muscle whenever it is put to use, and eventually becomes able to hold it under the control of his will, either exerting or relaxing his accommodation at pleasure.

In making the examination he should imagine that the retina is at least 100 yards away and should make every effort to keep his mind and accommodation upon that distance. If he will persist in this he will soon be successful and the retina will swim into view with the arteries, optic disc, etc., clear and distinct. It is usually the case that when the pupil has by persistent effort succeeded in relaxing his accommodation, thereby obtaining a distinct image for the first time, his attention is attracted away from the effort to relax, and in his desire to examine the retina he accommodates, when the image immediately vanishes again. As soon as he can once more relax, the retina once more comes before him, appearing and vanishing until he is successful in holding the accommodation back for an indefinite length of time. As stated above this requires patient and constant practice, but you can eventually master it.

In making this examination then we seat our patient with a lamp or gas flame directly behind his right shoulder, the optician seating himself at the right side of the patient with his chair facing the lamp. The patient being directed to look toward the farther end of the room, the optician places his ophthalmoscope before his own right eye and throwing the light into the right eye of the patient gradually approaches until the ophthalmoscope is almost against the patient's face. It is necessary to do this for the lenses of the ophthalmoscope must be at just the same distance from the patient's eye that spectacles will be worn, or the examination will prove inaccurate. He now turns his attention to the retina at the same time holding his accommodation perfectly at rest. If the patient's eye is emmetropic the retina will appear plain and distinct, if not it will be indistinct and he must turn the disc to find the correcting glass. If a plus glass is turned on and the retina appears more distinct, he continues to increase the convex power until he obtains the best possible view, adjusting his instrument by turning the disc, very much as one would adjust an opera-glass by turning the screw. The lens used in obtaining this distinct vision is the correcting glass of the patient. If with the plus glass the retina had appeared more indistinct, he would of course have turned to the minus, the one giving distinct vision being the measure of the myopia.

It is also necessary in this examination that the patient's eye be free from accommodation else the test will be incorrect. We cannot teach the patient to relax, nor is it always convenient to use drugs, but fortunately it has been found that with the intense light which is thrown into the eye during examination the accommodation usually gives up trying to act and remains passive. In fact one of the greatest advantages of the direct method is that the accommodation will generally relax more under this test than in any of the subjective tests. The Objective Examination may be summed up in the following rule. Copy:

95. In the Direct Method of Examination the observer must be an emmetrope, either naturally or artificially, with his accommodation at rest. The examination is made with the observer's eye very close to the patient's eye, and the lenses in the ophthalmoscope turned on until a distinct view of the retina is attained, the observer's eye being in a state of perfect rest. The number of the glass used is the correcting glass of the patient, unless astigmatism is present.

In examining the left eye, the observer sits on the left side of the patient looking through the instrument with his left eye. The test is made the same as for the right.

The Indirect Method.

In making the indirect examination the optician sits with his face about twenty inches from the patient and holds a strong convex lens (about 13 D) in front of the patient's eye. In this position he places the ophthalmoscope before his eye and turning his attention to the patient, examines the retina as it appears through the strong glass. Let us consider the action of rays proceeding from the retina under these conditions.

If the eye is emmetropic we know that rays coming from any point of the retina will emerge parallel. These parallel rays coming in contact with the convex glass will be brought to a focus at the principal focus of the glass, between the glass and the optician. There will then be a real inverted image of the retina in the air at the principal focus of the lens. Hartridge Fig. 37 shows rays coming from two different points of the optic disc (entrance of the optic nerve), each sending out its group of parallel rays which form an inverted image in the air at "ba." It is this aerial image that the optician really sees, for the rays must all cross at that place, and after crossing will diverge and come to the eye exactly as though the image were the original object. Of course the eye should accommodate for that particular point in order to see the image distinctly, but as this is difficult to do without considerable practice it will be fully as correct to turn up a plus 2.50 or 3.50 in the ophthalmoscope which will take the place of the required accommodation. The optician can then look directly into the eye for the optic disc, which is what he naturally would do. Now if he will gradually draw the convex lens away from the patient's eye toward his own, all the time keeping the optic disc in view, he will notice that the disc remains of exactly the same size at all times. This is easily explained by a glance at Hartridge Fig. 40, which represents the lens in two positions, one close to the eye, the other withdrawn a short distance. The emergent rays being parallel the image will always be the same and situated at the principal focus of the lens, moving along exactly with the lens. By this we know that the eye is emmetropic.

In the hypermetropic eye the rays will leave diverging and will come to a focus beyond the principal focus of the lens. (See Hartridge Fig. 38). The rays leaving the eye are just diverging enough to make them appear to have come from the points a and b back of the eye, and we must therefore consider this negative punctum remotum as the object. We have then our object at ab, our convex lens at c, and our image at ba. We have certainly studied lenses enough to know that if the lens is drawn away from the object, thus placing the object at a greater distance from it, the image will decrease in size and move toward the principal focus. It is upon this fact that we base our judgment of hypermetropia in the indirect examination. The optician fixes his attention upon the optic disc of the patient and gradually withdraws the convex lens. If the disc appears to decrease in size we know the eye to be hypermetropic.

In the myopic eye the rays will leave converging and will come to a focus between the convex lens and its principal focus (Hartridge Fig. 39). This focus ba is really the image of the virtual object at the left end of the diagram, for it is at that place that the rays would have met had they not been intercepted by the lens. The nearer to the virtual object the lens is brought, the larger will be the image ba, until the object is reached, when the image and object will be of the same size. In making the indirect examination in myopia therefore, a view of the optic disc is obtained, and if upon drawing the convex lens toward the optician's eye the disc appears to increase in size we know the eye to be myopic. The indirect examination may be summed up in the following rule. Copy:

> 96. *In the Indirect Method of Examination the observer sits about twenty inches from the patient looking through the plus 2.50 lens of his ophthalmoscope and examines the optic disc through a strong convex lens (about 13 D) held close to the patient's eye. If upon moving the lens away from the observed eye toward his own the disc appears to grow smaller the case is one of hypermetropia; if larger, myopia; if it remains the same size, emmetropia. The retina and disc as seen by the indirect method are always inverted.*

Concave Mirror at a Distance.

In making this examination the optician sits about twenty inches from the patient and examines the eye through the open hole of the ophthalmoscope, the strong convex lens not being used. If the eye is emmetropic it will be difficult to distinguish the retina distinctly. The reason for this is that the retina is situated at the principal focus of the eye and the rays leave parallel. Hartridge Fig. 43 shows the direction of these rays, one group from the point B of the retina going off parallel to one another toward D, and another group from the point A going off toward C. If the optician's eye is situated as far back as D or C it would be impossible to get rays from the two extremes of the disc or an artery as they have separated to such an extent. Of course if the optician was closer he would catch the rays before separating, but in that case he would be making the direct examination.

If upon looking into the eye, the retina with its arteries and optic disc are plainly seen, we know that it is not emmetropic but is either hypermetropic or myopic, for as shown in Fig. 44, the diverging rays from different points of the hypermetropic retina will over-lap one another in such a way that at all times rays from different points may be received, thus giving a distinct image. In myopia the rays leave converging but soon cross and diverge, giving the same distinct view as in hypermetropia. The image of the retina however is inverted in myopia on account of the rays crossing one another. To determine whether the defect is hypermetropia or myopia the optician fixes his attention upon one of the arteries and slowly moves his head from side to side. If the eye is hypermetropic the artery will appear to move in the same direction as the optician's head. This is easy to understand. Make a hole about one inch in diameter in a sheet of paper and draw a vertical line with your pencil on another sheet. Now lay the second sheet upon the table and look at the line through the hole in the first sheet, which you hold in your hand a couple of inches above the table. Now slowly move your head to the left and the line will appear to have also moved to the left, not because it has actually moved, but because the left edge of the hole is now between your eye and the line. Move your head over to the right and the line will appear to travel over in that direction and will disappear behind the right edge of the hole. It is this same movement which takes place when an artery is viewed through the pupil of a hypermetropic eye. The retina being between the crystalline lens and its principal focus, the rays come out diverging and the image of the artery is upright. If the eye is myopic the rays from the artery will emerge converging and will come to a focus and cross before reaching the observer's eye. The image will therefore be inverted and every movement appear just contrary to what it actually is. The artery therefore will move to the right when the optician's head moves to the left, and left when he moves to the right. This is a very simple and easy method of determining the condition of the eye.

If you will take a convex lens, the stronger the better, and try the following experiment this method of examination may be made still more plain. The lens in an ordinary pair of reading spectacles or the large lens of a jeweler's eye-glass will do. Hold your lead pencil behind the lens in a vertical position and view it through the lens. The lens represents the crystalline lens of the eye and the pencil an artery on the retina. Now move your head slowly to the right and the pencil will also appear to move to the right. This is because the pencil is between the lens and the principal focus thus giving us an upright image, which is the case in hypermetropia. Next move the pencil backward from the lens, and a point will soon be reached where the pencil fills up the entire lens and you can make out neither form nor shape. This point is the principal focus and represents Emmetropia. If you move it still farther back (myopia) you will find that when you move your head to the right the pencil will appear to move to the left. This is only because the conjugate of the pencil is between your eye and the lens, and the rays cross at that point thus giving you an inverted image. It will take you but a moment to try this experiment and it will repay you well for your trouble. This method of examination may be summed up in the following rule. Copy:

97. In making the "Concave Mirror at a Distance" examination the observer sits about twenty inches from the patient looking through the open hole of his ophthalmoscope and looks for an artery on the patient's retina. If he cannot obtain a distinct view the eye is emmetropic. If he sees an artery distinctly he moves his head slowly from side to side, and if the artery appears to move in the same direction it is hypermetropia. If in the opposite direction, myopia.

Retinoscopy, or the Shadow Test.

Retinoscopy, (also called Skiascopy, Pupilloscopy, or Koroscopy) consists of determining the refractive condition of an eye by watching the movements of light and shadows inside the eye as we pass a reflection over the eye. An instrument called the Retinoscope is used, which is similar to an ophthalmoscope except that there are no lenses and the concave mirror is larger. In fact it simply consists of a concave mirror with a hole in the center, and mounted on a handle. The examination is made similar to the ophthalmoscopic tests, except that the optician sits one meter in front of the patient. By throwing the light into the patient's eye, and looking through the sight-hole a red glow called "the fundus reflex" is seen through the pupil, simply from the fact that the retina is illuminated. Now if the mirror is turned a little to one side as if to move the light out of the eye, it will be seen that this reflex also moves on out of the pupil toward one side of the other, or what is more noticeable, a dark shadow which bounds the illumination will be seen to appear at one edge of the pupil and travel over to the other edge leaving the pupil dark. Sometimes this shadow moves in one direction sometimes in another, according as the eye is hypermetropic or myopic. This is a very simple and easy method of examination and at the same time one of the most important and accurate that we have.

In the case of small children and others who do not give us correct answers in the subjective tests, we can readily with a little practice, arrive at almost the exact condition of the eye by this method. The principles of retinoscopy however, and the reasons for the different shadow movements, are more difficult to understand than to make the tests. Let us consider the action of rays under these circumstances.

In Hartridge Fig. 52, "b" represents the flame, "a" the retinoscope and "c" the crystalline lens of the patient. Rays leave the flame, come in contact with the mirror and come to a focus at the conjugate between "a" and "c." Here they cross and of course are now inverted as they continue to approach the lens. Passing through the lens a focus is again reached which is now upright for we know that a convex lens always gives us an inverted image, and as the rays were already turned over by the mirror the lens will of course right them again. We therefore have an upright image of the flame on the line "e." Now if the mirror is turned a little to one side the image behind the lens will move in the opposite direction. This will always be the case whether the eye is hypermetropic, myopic or emmetropic. If hypermetropic the image is upon the retina nearer the principal focus, and we will see the movements as they actually take place. Therefore in hypermetropia the light and its surrounding shadow will be seen to move in the opposite direction to the mirror. In myopia however, the retina is behind the principal focus of the lens and the emerging rays will come to a focus and cross before they reach the optician's eye thus inverting every movement. Instead of moving opposite to the mirror, which is what they in reality do, they will APPEAR to move in the same direction.

The only exception to this rule is when the myopia is of less than 1 D. In that case the rays will reach the observer's eye before coming to a focus and will of course show the movements as they actually exist, for you will remember that the observer is one meter from the patient. Hartridge therefore says that if the shadow moves against the mirror the case is either one of hypermetropia, emmetropia or low myopia. This is somewhat confusing and to avoid complications I have in my practice hit upon the plan of placing before the patient's eye in the trial frame a plus 1 D glass which just neutralizes the distance at which I sit. By this plan I am enabled to say that when the shadow moves against the mirror the case is one of hypermetropia, and when with the mirror one of myopia. If the patient is emmetropic the light will seem to appear and disappear from both sides of the pupil at once, so that it will be impossible to distinguish any movement in either direction, except that the pupil is either entirely lighted up or not at all. This is because the emmetropic retina is at the principal focus of the dioptric system and the rays all come out parallel in a solid beam from all parts of the pupil as long as there is any light left within the eye.

To determine the degree of the defect we first place a convex lens of one dioptre before the patient's eye and look through the retinoscope at the reflex. If the light and shadow move in the opposite direction to the mirror, the case is one of hypermetropia and we put another convex lens in the frame with a view to making him emmetropic, continuing to add the lenses until the pupil lights up at once and there is no movement. If the shadow moves in the same direction we use concave lenses instead, stopping when we reach emmetropia. We now remove the plus 1 D lens which neutralized our distance and the remaining lenses constitute the correcting glass. Retinoscopy may be summed up in the following rule. Copy:

> 98. *In Retinoscopy the examination is made at a distance of one meter from the patient, and the red reflex in the eye together with the shadow bounding it is what we consider. Turning the mirror from side to side so that light passes across the eye we note in which direction the reflex and shadow moves. If they move in the same direction as the mirror the case is myopic. If the whole pupil is lighted up at once it is emmetropic. If they move in the opposite direction it is hypermetropic provided always that we have a plus 1 D lens before the eye of the patient to neutralize the 1 meter distance at which we stand. We now find the lens which will cause the pupil to be lighted up at once after which we remove the plus 1 D. The remaining lens is the correction of his Ametropia.*

For your study between mails take the sixth chapter of Hartridge.

QUESTIONS ON LESSON NO. 10.

161. How many methods of examination with the ophthalmoscope have we?
162. Explain briefly the principle of the Direct method?
163. Of the Indirect method?
164. Of the "Concave Mirror at a Distance."
165. What is Retinoscopy?
166. In what manner is the test made?
167. Why, in the "Concave Mirror" test, does the artery move the same direction as the head in Hypermetropia, while in Retinoscopy the light moves in the opposite direction?
168. Why does the optic disc appear to grow smaller in hypermetropia in the Indirect Examination?
169. Why is the glass through which we see best in the Direct Examination the correcting glass of the patient?

EXPLANATIONS ON LESSONS NO. 9 AND NO. 10.

151. Any examination of the eye in which we depend upon the sensations and judgement of the patient for our diagnosis. (*Rule 85.*)

152. Any examination of the eye in which we depend upon ourselves and what we see, for our diagnosis, without questioning the patient. (*Rule 86.*)

153. Give the patient the strongest plus lens through which he can still see his best line just as well as without. (*Rule 88.*)

154. Give the patient the weakest minus lens through which he is enabled to read his best line. (*Rule 89*).

155. We mean that the retina is only one-half as sensitive to light as the average retina.

In other words, the letter which can be read by the average retina twelve meters away must be brought to within six meters in order to be distinguished.

156. We mean that the eye has an AVERAGE retina. That is, when the rays are thrown to a focus upon it, it can distinguish objects at the distance that the average eye can distinguish them. Do not form the habit of calling this "normal" vision, for it is only an average found by taking the vision of many thousand normal eyes and striking an average of the whole. Many normal eyes see better and many worse than this. Also do not form the habit of in any way connecting 6/6 with emmetropia, for they have no relation whatever. Emmetropia refers to the position of the principal focus while 6/6 refers to the sensitiveness of the retina. In fitting glasses we do not give the strongest plus or weakest minus through which the patient can read 6/6 but through which he can read "his best." His best depends upon his retina entirely.

157. The pin-hole test tells us beyond a doubt whether the low vision is on account of the focus not being upon the retina, or from some other cause. In other words it tells us WHETHER THE FOCUS IS UPON THE RETINA OR NOT. The principle of the test is based upon the diagram on page 3 of Lesson No. 1, the candle representing the test type, the card H the pin-hole disc and the second card the retina. No matter where the retina is placed in the eye, and no matter whether there is even a crystalline lens in the eye or not, there will be an outline image of the test type thrown upon it and the patient will be able to discern the letters if his retina is a good one. If he is an emmetrope the focus is already upon the retina and the vision will not be improved by the pin-hole. Hence if he sees better through the pin-hole it tells us that the focus is NOT upon the retina. If he sees no better through the pin-hole the focus IS upon the retina. In other words, if he sees better through the pin-hole he is not an emmetrope. If he sees no better he is not a myope. In the latter case he is either an emmetrope of a hypermetrope for either of these two may have the focus upon the retina, the emmetrope naturally and the hypermetrope by his accommodation. The chief use of the pin-hole then is to reduce the condition to one of two defects which simplifies our work. It does not necessarily imply a disease, for low vision may be due to the fact that the rods and cones are placed farther apart than in the average eye and hence require larger images.

158. Cover one eye, ask patient to read his best line, hold up plus 0.25 D and ask him if he sees JUST AS WELL, if not, remove it and hold up minus 0.25 D and ask him if he sees BETTER. If so, leave it in the trial frame and hold up another minus 0.25 D asking the same question. If this is also better, exchange the two for minus 0.50 D (an even exchange which should be made quickly and without exposing the eye) and then add another minus 0.25 D asking the same question. If still better, exchange the two for 0.75 D and proceed as before until he finally says that vision is not better but about the same. Do not give him this last lens but stop at the last one that was a real improvement. Go through the same process with the other eye, then remove the blank disc and with the correction before each eye hold up plus 0.25 D in each hand and ask him if he sees JUST AS WELL. If so reduce each minus lens that much and try again, giving the weakest through which he sees his best.

159. Cover one eye, ask patient to read his best line, hold up plus 0.25 D and ask him if he sees JUST AS WELL. If so put on another 0.25 D and ask the same question. If so, exchange the two for 0.50 D and hold up 0.25 D again with the same question. Continue in

this manner as long as he accepts them. Do the same with the other eye and then with both eyes try still stronger giving him the strongest through which he sees at his best. Be very particular to use the question JUST AS WELL whenever you apply a plus lens and the question BETTER whenever you apply a minus lens.

160. I think this is fully covered on the sixth page of Lesson No. 9.

161. Three. The Direct, Indirect and Concave Mirror at a distance.

162.-163.-164.-165.-166. *Rules 95, 96, 97 and 98* really answer these questions as well as I could answer them again.

167. In the reflex test we are looking at a reflection of the lamp which has been thrown into the patient's eye by our concave mirror. The rays on their way from the mirror to the patient must, of course, cross at the focus of the mirror. Hence the reflection which we throw upon his retina is inverted and every movement will be a reserved movement. In the artery test we are looking at an artery which is already in the eye and upright. We do not throw this artery into the eye with our mirror. As it is upright we see the movement with us, not reversed.

168. As the rays come from the Hypermetropic eye as if they had come from his negative P. R. the object, so far as the strong convex lens is concerned, is really situated at the P. R. As we learned in Lesson No. 5 the greater the distance from the lens to the object, the smaller the image. Of course, in this case, drawing the lens from the eye increases its distance from the object. Hence the image decreases in size. In all conditions we may consider the P. R. of the eye as the object in the indirect method. In a myope the P. R. being in front of the eye, drawing the lens from the eye decreases the distance between the object and lens, hence the image increases in size. In emmetropia, as the P. R. is at infinity, the distance makes no appreciable difference, the rays being parallel at all distances.

169. As the optician is an emmetrope with no accommodation, the only eye into which he can see distinctly is an emmetropic eye. Hence the glass which enables him to clearly see the patient's retina, must be the glass which makes the patient emmetropic.

L E S S O N   N O.   11.

Hypermetropia.

NOT ONLY SHOULD we be competent to make the different tests for ametropia, but a thorough understanding of the symptoms, causes, effects and treatment of the different refractive conditions is indispensable. In this lesson we shall consider hypermetropia in its several phases and degrees, together with some of the anomalies which influence it.

Hypermetropia, or Hyperopia, is that condition of the eye in which the principal focus of the dioptric system is situated behind the retina. This may be due to one of three causes. (1) The eye may be too short on its antero-posterior axis, that is from front to back, which we call "Axial Hypermetropia"; (2) the convexity of the crystalline lens or cornea may be too slight, the length of the eye being normal, which we call "Curvature Hypermetropia"; or, (3) the index of refraction of the aqueous humor or crystalline lens may be less or that of the vitreous more than normal, which we call "Hypermetropia from change in the Index of Refraction." Sometimes it may be due to two or all of these causes combined. Whatever the cause we know that the principal focus is behind the retina and it is our business as opticians to move it forward to the yellow spot at the same time placing our patients under the most comfortable conditions possible.

Hypermetropia may be considered as an under-development of the eye, and is often associated with a marked under-development of the face and head. The eyes of children are as a rule hypermetropic, only reaching emmetropia as they grow older and all the portions of the body acquire full development. The eyes of the lower animals are nearly always hypermetropic. Indians and the uncivilized nations also show a hypermetropic tendency.

In considering the symptoms of our patients we should first note the face and general appearance of the eyes. In hypermetropia the eyes are usually small, sometimes deeply set in the orbits and are quick and restless in their movements owing to the strong leverage which the recti muscles have upon so small an eye. If you will cultivate this habit of studying the features and eyes of every patient you will soon be able to decide very accurately the refractive condition before proceeding to make the test. Next we should inquire in what way the eyes give trouble, listening to the patient's history of the case, which will always aid us in correctly diagnosing the existing defects. In hypermetropia, if it is of a moderate degree, say of less than 4 D or 5 D, the patient will likely say that his eyes tire and burn and sometimes water if he attempts to read for any length of time, and that the letters will blur and run together; or he may say that he has headaches almost constantly, or some other symptoms of irritation and over-work. These symptoms are given the name of "Asthenopia" which means a feeling of fatigue, pain or irritation from extra effort. The reason for asthenopia in hypermetropia may be traced to two causes: First, the patient is always compelled to use an extra amount of accommodation in order to overcome his hypermetropia, this overwork especially in reading or looking at near objects, becoming very tiresome; Second, the harmony between accommodation and convergence is disturbed, the patient being compelled at all times to use his accommodation a certain amount in excess of the effort of convergence. The latter I consider the most frequent cause of Asthenopia in the moderate degrees of hypermetropia, for we have many cases in which the patient has strong accommodation, certainly enough to comfortably handle one or two dioptres of excessive work, but who are victims of Asthenopia as a result of one-half or one-quarter dioptre of hypermetropia. This must certainly be due to the disturbed harmony between convergence and accommodation as the correcting glasses give them immediate and permanent relief.

In the higher degrees of hypermetropia the symptoms are very different. In these cases the patient, unless very young, does not have sufficient amplitude of accommodation to overcome his hypermetropia and therefore gives up trying to obtain distinct retinal images, and contents himself with circles of diffusion. In this way he would avoid all strain and overwork of the muscles of either accommodation or convergence, so that he suffers no asthenopia, and at the same time escapes strabismus. His only complaint is that he cannot see well even at a distance. This of course stimulates myopia making it difficult to determine between the two so far as we judge by symptoms. The symptoms in reading are also similar to myopia, the patient being obliged to hold the book very close to his eyes. The reason for this is that although he at all times receives only circles of diffusion upon the retina, the visual angle is much larger when the object is brought close to the eye, so that the diffusion spreads out over a larger portion of the retina and enables him to distinguish the form and outline of the letters. In those cases of high degree hypermetropia there the patient has enough accommodation to overcome the defect, if they make the effort and do so they will certainly acquire the habit of strabismus providing the accommodation is used beyond the limit of relative accommodation.

Spasm of Accommodation.

Very frequently the cilliary muscles of an eye through over-work or irritation takes upon itself a spasmodic or contracted condition from which it is powerless to free itself. No doubt you have many times experienced a spasm or "cramp" in the muscles of the arm, or limb which is extremely painful. You could contract the muscles as much as you wished but could not straighten it beyond a certain limit. This is just what takes place in the cilliary muscle in these cases of accommodative spasm. The muscle is free to exert itself as much as ever but cannot entirely relax. Spasm of the accommodation very frequently lasts for years beginning in the child and lasting until gradual loss of accommodation by age at last compels it to give up. This condition is very frequent in hypermetropes owing to the excessive work which the accommodation is compelled to do. In fact we must always watch for this condition in every case we have for it is a very common one.

What effect will spasm of accommodation have upon the Hypermetropic eye? The principal focus of this eye is behind the retina. A spasm of the cilliary muscles will of course increase the convexity of the crystalline lens thus bringing rays to a focus quicker and therefore nearer the retina so that the hypermetropia appears to be of less degree than it really is. Should the spasm be of sufficient intensity the focus may be brought to the retina making the eye appear emmetropic, or it may even bring it past the retina making the eye myopic. This condition therefore renders it very difficult to determine whether the glasses we prescribe are the correct ones or not. The hypermetropia may be one of 4 D while the strongest glass he will accept may be a plus 2.00, plus 1.00, or he may refuse the weakest plus glass or even read better with a minus glass owing to the spasm of accommodation which will not allow the cilliary muscle to relax. We must therefore be very careful that we do not underestimate the refractive condition. In the case of high spasm we are very likely to find what we take to be a slight myopia and to prescribe minus lenses when we really have a case of hypermetropia. The minus lenses will only act as an encouragement to the spasm making it necessary for the cilliary muscle to exert itself at all times to that amount in order to see at all, so that instead of relieving the excessive work of the muscle, we have provoked it to greater action which will very likely cause greater spasm.

How may we detect and overcome such a condition? To describe the symptoms which lead us to suspect it is difficult. It is only by experience and a knowledge of the symptoms in different conditions that we are enabled to determine its existence. For instance, if we have a case apparently myopic, but with all the symptoms of hypermetropia, we at once suspect spasm. If a patient shows hypermetropia, and in making the examination we find he will at times accept a certain plus lens while at other times he will not, the accommodation appearing variable and unstable, we at once decide that spasm exists. Again if a low degree of hypermetropia shows severe asthenopic symptoms which naturally belong to higher degrees we are led to look for spasm. The condition is a very common one in young people but of course rare in people of advanced age owing to diminution in the power of accommodation.

There is but one thorough and complete method of overcoming spasm of accommodation and that is by the use of a mydriatic. A mydriatic is any drug which has the power of temporarily paralyzing the cilliary muscle thereby depriving it of all power to act. Atropine, (or atropia) is the most active mydriatic which we possess and is most used by oculists. It contains the active principle of Belladonna. Homatropine is a quicker mydriatic and the effects pass off much sooner, but it is not so thorough. It is used however by a great many. By the use of a mydriatic the cilliary muscle is compelled to give up its effort and remain passive thus completely overcoming the spasm of accommodation and we can then measure the eye accurately, and know that we are determining the actual defect. You will notice that many authors recommend mydriatics in nearly every case, especially if the patients are young. Hartridge speaks of atropizing his patients in nearly every test which he describes. This is of course good theory but is hardly practicable in our everyday work, as the patient is obliged to undergo considerable inconvenience while the effect of the mydriatic lasts. We will therefore in our practice as opticians, confine the atropine treatment to those cases of marked spasm of accommodation where the symptoms indicates a strong necessity for it. In the ordinary cases I follow the plan of giving the hypermetrope a full correction of the defect which he shows during the test, requesting him to wear the glasses and return in a few days for another examination. The chances are that he will then show a higher degree of hypermetropia, some of the spasm having disappeared owing to the relief from excessive work obtained by the glasses. I can now increase the strength of his lenses, continuing to do so every few days until the spasm disappears. In those cases which require the use of mydriatic I would suggest that you have an understanding with some physician of your place and that you refer the patient to him to obtain the medicine and prescription. He can charge them his regular office fee for his service and you will be the gainer in having his good will and influence, for the physicians of a place are the most powerful friends the optician has. You may depend upon his reciprocating many times over by sending you customers that will pay you much better money than any you ever send him. It is decidedly unwise for the optician to do his own prescribing for not only is such an offense punishable by law, but the influence of the physician is also lost.

The use of mydriatics not only relaxes the accommodation fully but dilates the pupils to a considerable extent. It is a good plan for either the physician or yourself to explain to the patient just what to expect so that he will not become alarmed after using the medicine. Tell him that the pupils will become dilated and if hypermetropic his vision will be very poor, for you know that if the power to accommodate is taken from him he will be unable to move his focus up to the retina. His vision for near will of course be worse. It is well for him to wear smoked glasses while the pupil is dilated to shut out some of the excessive light, and you may give him a pair of convex glasses to take the place of his accommodation when reading. The treatment should last three days, dropping one drop of the solution in each eye after each meal. He then comes to you for examination after which he will not need to continue the use of the mydriatic. It will usually take about a week for the effects to pass away. In fitting eyes which are under the influence of a mydriatic, it is always necessary to deduct 0.25 D from the result. The reason for this is, that the mydriatic rather over-does the matter and relaxes the accommodation about 0.25 more than it would naturally rest. In hypermetropia the mydriatic would show 0.25 D more of the defect than really exists, and myopia 0.25 D less than the actual defect. Thus if an eye under atropine shows 2 D of hypermetropia we say he is 1.75 D hypermetropic, and if it shows 2 D of myopia we know him to have 2.25 D. Copy:

99. *Spasm of accommodation is a cramped condition of the cilliary muscle which renders it impossible to relax beyond a certain limit. It makes Hypermetropia less hypermetropic, emmetropic or even myopic; Emmetropia appear myopic; and Myopia appear more myopic.*

100. *Spasm of accommodation may be relieved by the use of mydriatics which temporarily paralize the cilliary muscle and at the same time dilate the pupil. Atropia and Homatropine are most frequently used.*

101. *In fitting eyes which are under the influence of mydriatics it is always necessary to allow a difference of 0.25 D for the over effect of the drug. In hypermetropia we subtract that amount from the result found, and in myopia we add.*

———————o◯o———————

Spasm of accommodation producing different effects upon the hypermetropic eye has made it necessary to divide Hypermetropia into two classes: Manifest and Latent. Copy:

> *102. Manifest Hypermetropia is that hypermetropia which is readily revealed by the test.*
>
> *103. Latent Hypermetropia is that hypermetropia which is hidden by spasm of accommodation, the spasm making it impossible for the cilliary muscle to relax.*
>
> *104. The sum of the manifest and latent hypermetropia is called the "Total Hypermetropia."*
>
> *105. Manifest Hypermetropia is divided into two classes. Facultative and Absolute.*
>
> *106. Facultative Hypermetropia is that which the eye has sufficient accommodative power to overcome, thus seeing equally as well as the emmetrope.*
>
> *107. Absolute Hypermetropia is that which he has not the power to overcome, his focus remaining behind the retina in spite of his efforts to move it forward.*

For instance let us suppose that the patient shows a manifest hypermetropia of 3 D, and that he shows an amplitude of accommodation of only 1 D. It will be impossible for him to see distinctly even at infinity, for his accommodation is not sufficiently strong to bring the focus up to the retina. If we give him a plus of 2.00 D lens however, he will be able to overcome the remaining 1 D by the use of his accommodation. His manifest hypermetropis is therefore divided into 2D of absolute and 1D of facultative. Let us also suppose that we have reasons to suspect a spasm of the accommodation and send him to a physician for atropine. At the end of three days he once more returns and we find that the only glass with which he sees well is a plus 4.50 D. This shows us that there was on the previous day, some latent hypermetropia which has now become manifest. Allowing 0.25 D for the atropine he has now 4.25 D of manifest hypermetropia, all of which is absolute, as his accommodation is powerless to act. We can say then that at the first accommodation is powerless to act. We can say then that at the first examination he had 1.25 D of latent and 3 D of manifest hypermetropia, the latter being divided into 2 D of absolute and 1 D of facultative. His total hypermetropia therefore is 4.25 D and his amplitude of accommodation 2.25 D instead of 1 D which he appeared to have on the first day.

Having determined by the different subjective and objective tests, the exact condition of our hypermetrope what shall we prescribe for his correction? Naturally you would answer that the full amount of his defect should be corrected. Theoretically this is true but in practical work we must be more conservative. Hypermetropes of strong accommodative power will hardly bear a full correction, for the old habit of accommodating for every distance still remains and is very difficult to break up, so that the patient will hardly thank you for the inconvenience which you have caused him. A good rule in hypermetropia is to give a correction of all the manifest and one-third to one-half the latent. This is in the ordinary cases. Of course in cases of children just forming the habit of strabismus it is important beyond everything else that the full amount of hypermetropia be overcome. In the lower degree of hypermetropia, say up to about 2 D in young persons whose only complaint is asthenopia, a full correction of the manifest to be worn only for reading and near work is sufficient, increasing the strength of the glass later if more of the defect becomes manifest. In the higher degrees of hypermetropia it is best that the patient wear his glasses constantly. The treatment of the different defects will be more thoroughly covered later, in the practical portion of the course. For the present what has already been said will suffice.

There still remains one other form of hypermetropia known as Aphakia. This is a condition in which the crystalline lens is absent and may be caused by injury, dislocation, or what is most frequently the case, a cataract operation. As the crystalline lens is usually equal in strength to from 10 D to 13 D, its absence must necessarily diminish the refraction of the eye to a considerable extent thus throwing the focus farther back, and, unless the patient was previously a myope of at least the same degree as the strength of the lens, hypermetropia will result. For instance if the eye was emmetropic and the lenses equal to a plus 11.00 we find after extraction that the eye is 11 D hypermetropic. If it was 3 D hypermetropic the removal of the lens will leave 14 D of hypermetropia; if 4 D myopic it will leave 7 D of hypermetropia and so on. A myope of just 11 D therefore would be rendered emmetropic by the operation, but I am afraid that the remedy would be "worse than the disease."

The removal of the lens of course destroys all accommodations so that the patient is in the same condition so far as the accommodation is concerned, as a person of 75 or 80 years of age. He must therefore have a lens for viewing distant objects and one for near work and reading. For instance if he requires a plus 12.00 for distance he will require a plus 15.00 for reading at 33 cm. Any other distances, as 50 cm or 20 cm would require still other lenses, but the patient usually forms the habit of sliding the spectacles farther down or higher up on his nose, thus in a measure adjusting his focus for slightly different distances. He must however have the two lenses, one for far and one for near.

As patients usually have but one eye operated upon for cataract, leaving the other blind, we can put up their glasses in what is known as "cataract frames." These consist of a pair of spectacles with the nose piece so shaped that they can be worn either side up. The distance lens is placed in one side and the lens for reading in the other, so that when one is before the aphakic eye the other is before the blind eye. When he wishes to change, he simply turns them over and the lenses change places. This saves the inconvenience of carrying two pairs of glasses.

Although Hartridge has very carefully covered the subject of Myopia, I think it will be well to devote one lesson to its study as we cannot understand these subjects too thoroughly. Before Lesson No. 12 arrives I would have you study over the seventh chapter of Hartridge very carefully, not only once but many times. I trust you do not neglect any of these studies between mails for they are very important.

(End of Lesson No. 11.)

QUESTIONS ON LESSON NO. 11.

170. Can we have a case 12D Hypermetropic without converging strabismus? If so under what condition does he see?

171. What are some of the symptoms of hypermetropia in a moderate degree?

172. What are some of its causes?

173. Describe the different tests for hypermetropia.

174. What is meant by spasm of the accommodation?

175. What effect may a spasm of accommodation have upon hypermetropia?

176. How many kinds of hypermetropia are there and what are they?

177. Suppose you have a patient in the chair who reads 6/18 without a glass; with a plus 1.50 he reads 6/6; with a plus 1.75 he reads 6/6; with a plus 2.00, 6/8. You send him to a physician for atropia and at the end of three days he reads best with a plus 3.75. State all the different kinds of hypermetropia which he had, on the first day and the amount of each.

178. What is Aphakia?

179. How can you determine the existence of aphakia?

180. What glass would you give a boy of 16 years who has 2 D of manifest hypermetropia, and 1 D of latent, and has been complaining of severe headaches?

181. Would you prescribe glasses for all the time or only for near work?

182. What are the symptoms in high degrees of hypermetropia?

183. What is Asthenopia?

LESSON NO. 12.

Myopia.

MYOPIA IS THAT condition of the eye in which the principal focus of the dioptric system is situated in front of the retina. As in hypermetropia it may be due to three causes. (1) The eye may be too long on its antero-postero axis, which we call "Axial Myopia"; (2) the convexity of the crystalline lens or cornea may be too great, which we call "Curvature Myopia"; or (3) the index of refraction of the aqueous humor crystalline lens may be greater, or that of the vitreous less, than normal, which we call "Myopia from change in the Index of Refraction." Again it may be due to two or all of these causes combined.

Hypermetropia being considered as an under-development of the eye, myopia on the other hand may be regarded as an abnormal or over-development, the face and head frequently showing a similar tendency. Children who are born hypermetropes often pass on in their development beyond the emmetropic line, into the myopic. The higher civilized nations show a much greater percent of myopia than the barbarous, owing, it is believed, to the tendency of nature to adapt us to the conditions in which we are placed. People in the civilized countries being called upon to perform a great deal of close work, as reading, writing, fine arts, manufacturing, etc., the eye naturally attempts to conform itself to the new conditions and in a generation or so, myopia is the result. A very high percent of the inhabitants of Germany are myopic, and people living in town and cities show a greater tendency to this defect than those living in the country, distant vision not being required to so great an extent.

The symptoms of myopia are: A full developed head and face, large prominent eyes which turn slowly in their orbits, imperfect vision for distance, with good vision for near. The patient will not likely complain of asthenopic symptoms except when reading, writing or sewing, for we know that when he looks at an infinite distance neither his accommodation nor convergence is in use, hence no strain. The only inconvenience is that he sees indistinctly. In looking at near objects however, he sees well but the convergence being in excess of his accommodation creates a strain which results in asthenopia. In the low degrees of myopia the patient will suffer less from these symptoms and will even see fairly well at a distance, a great many going through life without even discovering that vision is less than normal. Some of them even become skillful in target practice with the rifle, and are only barred from such occupations as naval duties, piloting, etc., which require keen vision at great distances. In the medium and higher degrees however, the distant vision is considerably lessened, and in reading, the book must be held very close to the eyes in order to be within the far point. The asthenopic symptoms are of course much more intense owing to the greater disturbance between accommodation and convergence, except in those cases of high myopia who give up the effort and obtain relief through divergent strabismus, and in another class of cases who form the habit of reading with but one eye. These two classes are not apt to complain of asthenopia. The pupils of young myopes are usually quite large, becoming smaller as age advances. A great many myopes form the habit of closing their lids nearly together when they wish to see something distinctly. The reason for this is that the lids shut out some of the diffused rays giving them only the central rays, upon the same principle as the pin-hole test.

Spasm of accommodation in myopia will make the defect appear greater than it really is. For instance a myope of 1 D having a spasm of 2 D might accept nothing short of a 3.00 D for best vision. We must therefore be very careful lest we give myopes too strong glasses, thus creating a still greater spasm of accommodation through the excessive work imposed upon them. From the effects produced by spasm of accommodation we may divide myopia into "Apparent" and "Real." Copy:

108. Myopia, owing to spasm of accommodation is divided into two classes, Apparent and Real.

109. Apparent Myopia is the total defect which the patient appears to have while under the test.

110. Real Myopia is that which he really possesses, shown when the spasm of accommodation is overcome.

Thus in the case cited above the apparent myopia was 3 D while the real myopia was 1 D. In using atropine we must make an allowance of 0.25 as stated in Lesson 11 for the over relaxation of the muscle. In myopia we must of course add the 0.25 D to the result found instead of subtracting, for the atropine has made the myopia appear to be that much less than it really is. Thus if upon the first test an apparent myopia of 2.50 D is shown, and under atropine the best vision is obtained with a − 1.50, we know that the real myopia is 1.75 D and that the spasm of accommodation amounted to 0.75 D.

In ordinary types of myopia the treatment consists of a full correction of the defect by concave glasses in the low and medium degrees, except in the case of older patients when a different glass must of course be given for reading in addition to the distance glasses. In the higher degrees however, even in young myopes, it will be doubtful if reading can be done with the distance glasses, thus making it necessary to give them weaker lenses for that purpose, the same as in the case of old people. The full correction is of course to be given for distance. The reason that these myopes are unable to read with the full correction is easy to understand. Take for instance a myope of 8 D. The most distant point at which he can see distinctly is 12½ cm (5 inches), and this is performed without any effort of accommodation. There is certainly never any occasion to see at a closer point than this, so it is evident that our patient has spent all his life without ever having used a single dioptre of accommodation. The cilliary muscle must therefore be in a weakened condition on the same principle as tying one's arm in a sling for several months would take all muscular tone from that member. When we put on the correcting glasses therefore, we have made an emmetrope of him and in order to read at the ordinary reading distance (33) cm he must now use 3 D of accommodation. This being the first call ever made upon his accommodative power is naturally very tiresome and more of an effort than he can well bear at first. It is advisable then that we give him a somewhat weaker glass for reading, which will relieve part of this work but still give him some work to do. In this way the weak muscles gradually become accustomed to the exercises so that little by little we can increase the strength of his reading glass, until in the course of a few weeks or months, he will be able to perform all the required work without help, and we may take his reading glasses from him, the full correction sufficing for all distances. In the case referred to (8 D myopia) I would advise — 8.00 for distance and about — 6 D for reading, advising him to call again in a week or two. This will give him but 1 D of accommodative work to do in reading at 33 cm. This he should be able to do for a short time at least. Advise him to stop reading whenever he feels that his eyes are becoming tired, and wait until another time. By reading a little several times a day the muscles will soon become stronger and we can change his glasses to perhaps — 6.50, and so on. This of course applies to patients under 45 years of age, as people above that age having lost a part of their accommodative powers will always be compelled to use separate glasses for reading.

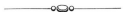

Thus far we have spoken of the regular, or typical forms of myopia. There remains one other form of this anomaly to be considered, a condition vicious in all its tendencies and deplorable in its results. I refer to what is known as "Progressive," "Pernicious," or "Malignant Myopia" which, as the name implies, is an ever increasing form of myopia, constantly becoming higher in degree from day to day.

Malignant Myopia is an evil which almost any myope is liable to take on at any time. The myopia may for years remain stationary, representing the ordinary types of the defect, when without a moment's warning it may some day take on the malignant form, the eye-ball becoming abnormal in growth, constantly increasing in length, breaking down the structure of the eye, and eventually resulting in partial or complete loss of sight. Let us consider the cause of this abnormal condition.

Myopes of the medium or higher degrees are compelled to bring their work or reading very close to the eyes in order to get the focus upon the retina. In other words they must bring the object not farther away than their punctum remotum. A myope of 5 D must be within 8 inches (20 cm) of the object before he can obtain distinct vision; one of 10 D within 4 inches (10 cm); and so on. Now if you will hold an object 5 or 6 inches in front of your friend's eyes asking him to look at it, you will see that his eyes are converging very strongly. In fact it is considerable of an effort for thim to maintain the position. This is what the myope must do in order to obtain binocular vision (single vision with both eyes at once) and when we remember that this convergence must be carried on in connection with the effort of holding back all accommodation, which is contrary to all natural tendency, you must know that the strain upon him is much greater than that imposed upon your friend when he looked at the near object. This effort of holding back the accommodation must, as we have seen in the lesson on convergence, create a corresponding desire upon the part of the eyes to lessen convergence which is only overcome by the will power of the individual. Thus we have a constant strain and tension of the recti muscles at all times when objects are held before the eyes for inspection.

What is the result of this tension upon the myopic eye? We know that the myope's eye is a long one and that the recti muscles coming from the back of the orbit, pass along the side of the eye-ball and attach themselves to it near the anterior portion. These muscles lying so closely along the eye must, when very strong tension is exerted during convergence, create a tremendous pressure upon the eye-ball. This pressure will cause the eye to give way sooner or later, and as the weakest point is at the optic disc, where the nerve penetrates through the choroid, that point will be the first to yield, and will be crowded or pushed backward toward the posterior portion of the orbit giving the optic disc a cupped or distended appearance, called a "Staphyloma." As the macula is but a short distance from the optic disc it is of course easy to understand that it, too, will share in the backward movement to a certain extent. This being the case the distance is of course greater from the cornea to the macula, and we have a higher degree of myopia than before, with a still greater tension upon the recti muscles. This of course only aggravates the pressure upon the eye-ball, and the optic disc and surrounding parts are crowded farther backward, once more creating a higher degree of myopia which in its turn creates greater pressure than ever before.

It is evident then that the condition will perniciously continue in its ruinous progression, until the posterior walls of the eye are stretched and distended to their utmost limit. Even here the trouble does not end, for the tension and pressure of the recti still continuing, the eye must give way still more. Accordingly the retina soon begins to give way becoming detached from the choroid in places, and tearing or becoming atrophied at other places. Gradually the macula becomes involved in the general ruin so that the patient loses direct vision and can only see indirectly as rays entering the eye from some object situated to one side of the visual line. Hemorrhages here and there begin to show themselves upon the retina, bleeding for a while, requiring a long time to heal again, and leaving blind spots when they do heal. The patient is harassed by black spots floating before the eyes, bright flashes of dazzling light when the eyes are closed, and an intolerance of light (photophobia), all conspire to make the poor victim's life miserable. He is frightened by imaginary terrors at every new sympton, the optic nerve becomes diseased, cataract often sets in, the vitreous humor becomes liquified, and if one eye is more diseased than the other it is likely to necessitate a removal of the bad eye in order to avoid a sympathetic disease in the better one. Both are usually bad enough.

On the plate opposite Page 147 in Hartridge is shown the retina in four different stages of malignant myopia. The first shows the white crescent on one edge of the optic disc, known as the "myopic crescent" which nearly always exists in the moderately high degrees of myopia. This is caused by a tendency to staphyloma which leaves this edge in a drawn state and soon becomes atrophied and insensible to light, eventually showing the white sclerotic through the thinned membranes. The other cuts represent conditions in more advanced stages, the white spot showing those portions of the retina which have become detached or atrophied.

As a preventative of malignant myopia, properly adjusted concave lenses are certainly valuable as they make it possible for the patient to hold his book or work at a normal distance, thus avoiding excessive convergence. In the first stages of progression concave lenses will at least retard, if not stop, the abnormal growth, but in the more advanced stages glasses are not of much effect. In fact the diseased condition of the eye renders the retina so extremely sensitive that it apparently cannot even bear distinct images, the correcting glasses producing intolerable pain. Very often I have had patients who, when the correcting glasses were placed before their eyes, would say: "That is delightful, I never saw so well before," but almost in the same breath would brush them aside, saying: "Oh I cannot bear them, they hurt my eyes." Of course in such cases it will be useless to prescribe a full correction, so if we attempt to give glasses at all it must only be what the patient can comfortably bear. I have a patient at present who is 11 D myopic, but who can only wear comfortably a − 4.50 D. In addition to these I have put a pair of − 5.50 D lenses in a grab-front frame (a frame made to hook over the regular glasses in such a way that the patient looks through both pairs.) This she is to use whenever she wishes to see some object distinctly for an instant, the two combined being equal to the full correction. Of course she can only keep them on for a moment, but they aid her considerably in getting occasional glimpses of distant objects.

In a great many cases complete rest and medical treatment are required rather than glasses, and I believe where it is practicable that the optician should refer the patient to some first-class oculist, for the patient's interests are much greater in importance than the occasional profit one might gain by prescribing lenses.

Measuring Lenses.

Very often a customer brings in a pair of glasses with one lens broken or cracked, which he wishes replaced. It is necessary that we know the strength of the lens in order that we may furnish a duplicate. There are many instruments upon the market, made with a view to measuring lenses, samples of which we find lying in dust upon the top shelf of nearly every jewelry store we enter. With the exception of perhaps one or two, these instruments are of no practical value, for while we can measure spherical lenses fairly well with them, they are worthless when we come to compound lenses. We have a much more simple, accurate, and inexpensive method of measuring all lenses, and that is by "neutralization." Let us study the principles of this method carefully, for it must be put to practical use every day.

First we wish to determine whether the lens is concave or convex. We know that concave lenses are thickest at the edge, while the convex are thickest at the center. A ray of light passing exactly through the optical center of either lens will pass straight on without refraction, but if it passes through any other portion it will be bent toward the thickest edge. Hence the object looked at will appear displaced to one side or the other if we look at through a lens at any point between its optical center and the edge. In the diagram, A represents a convex lens so placed that a ray coming from the ob-

ject O, passes through its optical center to the eye without deviation. B shows the same lens displaced in such a manner that the ray now passes through another portion, and is of course refracted toward the center. The ray coming to the eye in that direction will make the object appear to be at L. Thus the lens has been moved in one direction while the object apparently has been moved the opposite way. Copy: *MEASURING LENSES.—*

> *111. If an object is viewed through a lens, and upon moving the lens from side to side the object appears to move in the opposite direction, we know the lens to be convex.*

C shows a concave lens so placed that the ray passes through the optical center, while D shows the same lens displaced. This time the object appears to have moved in the same direction as the lens. Copy:

> *112. If an object is viewed through a lens, and upon moving the lens from side to side the object appears to move in the same direction, we know the lens to be concave.*

Having determined whether the lens is convex or concave, we next wish to ascertain the number, or strength. Diagram E shows us that parallel rays of light passing through a convex and concave lens of the same power will continue parallel, the positive power of one just neutralizing the negative power of the other, making the two equal to a plano lens. We have only to find the lens of opposite sign which will neutralize the given lens, in order to find its strength. To make this more clear let us suppose that a lens is given us to duplicate and we find upon moving it from side to side that the object looked at appears to move in the opposite direction. We know therefore that the lens is a convex one, and accordingly go to the concave lenses to look for a glass which will neutralize it. We take up for instance a − 1.00 D and look through the two lenses toward an object. Upon moving them from side to side we find that the object still appears to move in the opposite direction, so we know that our − 1.00 D is not strong enough. We next try a − 2.00 D and with this find that the object appears to

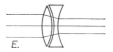

move in the same direction as the lenses. By this we know that the − 2.00 D is too strong, for it has not only overcome the convex power of the given lens but shows an excess of concave power. We must therefore try a lens somewhere between the − 1.00 D and − 2.00 D. Accordingly we select a − 1.50 D and with this the object still appears to move with the glass. With the − 1.25 D the object stands still, no movement taking place at all. This then is the neutralizing glass and we know that the lens we are measuring is a plus 1.25. If the lens had been a concave we would of course have looked for a convex lens of equal power to neutralize it. With a little practice one can sit down to the trial case and number lenses very rapidly.

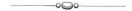

The examination with this lesson consists of a general review. Take plenty of time in writing your answers as it is important that all the points over which we have passed be thoroughly understood before taking up Astigmatism in Lesson No. 13. For your study between mails take the eighth chapter of Hartridge.

QUESTIONS ON LESSON NO. 12.

184. What is the visual angle and its uses?

185. Give the laws governing reflection.

186. What is the secondary axis of a concave mirror?

187. If an object is placed 40 cm in front of a 10-inch concave mirror, give relative size, position and location of image.

188. Will it be real or virtual?

189. Give description of image if the object is placed 15 cm from the same mirror.

190. If placed 25 cm from the mirror.

191. Where will you place an object before a concave mirror to get the smallest possible real image?

192. To get the largest possible real image?

193. To get the largest and the smallest virtual images?

194. Draw a diagram showing the course of rays coming from an arrow some distance from a convex mirror and showing where the image is produced.

195. Draw one with the arrow quite near the glass.

196. Why does a ray of light refract when passing obliquely from one medium to another, and why is it not refracted when passing perpendicularly?

197. Give the laws which tell us in which direction light will be refracted.

198. If we place an arrow one foot and eight inches from a plus 4.00 D lens give the size, position, location, etc., of the image.

199. If the arrow is placed 25 cm from the lens tell me about the image.

200. Draw a diagram showing the object, rays and image, the arrow being placed between the principal focus and secondary focus of a convex lens.

201. Draw one having the object between the principal focus and the convex lens.

202. Where will you place the object to get the smallest possible image with a concave lens, and where will the image be situated?

203. To get the largest possible image?

204. Give the focal distance in cm, of a plus 2.25 D lens.

205. What is the strength of a lens whose focal distance is 40 cm?

206. Of one whose focal length is 8 inches?

207. If you place a plus 1.50 D, a —3.25 D and a plus 0.25 D together, what is the strength of the combination?

208. Draw a rough diagram of the eye naming each part.

209. Name the muscles which control the movements of the eye.

210. What is the function of the superior obliques?

211. Of the inferior obliques?

212. What is accommodation?

213. What is the amplitude of accommodation of an eye whose punctum proximum is at 8 cm and whose punctum remotum is at 2 meters?

214. Where is the punctum remotum of an eye whose amplitude of accommodation is 7 D and whose punctum proximum is at 40 cm?

215. Explain relative convergence and relative accommodation.

216. Why does Hypermetropia sometimes cause converging strabismus?

217. How much convergence and how much accommodation is used by a 2.50 D myope in reading at 33 cm.
218. What is Chromatic Aberration, and how may it be overcome?
219. What is Spherical Aberration?
220. If the optician is a hypermetrope of 1.50 D and uses the ophthalmoscope without correcting himself, what is the correcting glass for the patient if it requires a —3.00 D to distinctly see the retina in the direct examination?
221. If the optician is 1 D myopic and it requires a plus 3.00 D lens?
222. If a patient shows a myopia of 3 D, and after using atropine reads best with a —2.25 D what is his real myopia?
223. What is Malignant Myopia?
224. What is the cause of Malignant Myopia?
225. How would you treat it?
226. How would you equip a 10 D myope (not malignant) age 24, who had never worn glasses?

EXPLANATIONS ON LESSONS NO. 11 AND NO. 12.

170. If he accommodates to bring his focus to the retina, the convergence will also act and he will be cross eyed. If he finds the effort too great for comfort and refused to accommodate the convergence will not be called upon and he will not be cross eyed. Of course he will see very indistinctly for the focus is behind the retina. He will however be comfortable and will escape strabismus.

171. Good vision for distance and near. Eyes tire in reading. Sometimes headaches or other asthenopic symptoms. As the hypermetrope is only moderate there will be no facial symptoms apparent.

172. The eye too short from front to back; the curvature of the cornea or lens too slight; the aqueous or lens of too great density, or the vitreous too rare.

173. The trial case test (the most important of all) in which we give the strongest plus lens through which the patient can still see just as well as without. The direct method in which we use the strongest plus through which we can see the retina distinctly. The indirect method in which the disc grows smaller as we draw the strong plus lens towards us. The concave mirror at a distance in which the artery appears to move with us. The retinoscope in which the reflex moves against us when a concave mirror is used and with us if a plane mirror is used.

174. A cramped condition of the cilliary muscle in which it cannot relax to the utmost although it can exert itself to as great a degree as when the spasm is not present.

175. As he cannot entirely relax the focus remains farther forward than is natural and the test therefore shows less hypermetropia than actually exists. The spasm may be so great as to leave the focus upon the retina or in front of it, thus making the eye test emmetropic or myopic.

176. Total hypermetropia which is divided into Latent and Manifest, the latter being sub-divided into Absolute and Facultative.

177. The fact that without a glass he did not read his best line tells us that the focus is not upon the retina. We find that we are obliged to add plus lenses until we have reached 1.50 D before he sees at his best. This then must be the part of his hypermetropia that he could not overcome himself. In other words it is absolute. We now add 0.25 more and he

sees just as well. This must be because he was accommodating and has relaxed that amount. We try another quarter making 2 D in all and he refuses it so we must go back to the 1.75 D. This, according to *Rule 88*, is his manifest hypermetropia, divided, as we have seen into 1.50 D of absolute and 0.25 D of facultative. Under atropine he shows 3.75 D of hypermetropia, which, after deducting 0.25 D for over effect of the drug, shows a total hypermetropia of 3.50 D. As his manifest is 1.75 D we have by deducting the manifest from the total, a latent of 1.75 D. Answer: Total 3.50, Latent 1.75, Manifest 1.75. Absolute 1.50. Facultative 0.25 D. We can also find the amplitude of accommodation in this case by subtracting the absolute (that which he has not the accommodation to overcome) from the total hypermetropia which leaves the amount that he DID overcome.

178. That condition in which the crystalline lens is absent.

179. Hartridge's plan of judging by the images formed when holding a light in front of, and a little to one side of the eye is the best answer to this question.

180. The rule in such cases is to correct all of the manifest and one-half of the latent, so I would prescribe plus 2.50 D.

181. This is hypermetropia of sufficiently high a degree to give trouble even for distant vision, for without glasses he would be compelled to accommodate at least 3 D wherever he looked when upon the street. I would therefore have him wear the glasses constantly.

182. If he accommodates to overcome the defect he will be cross eyed. If not, then his eyes will be at rest but he will see very indistinctly. He will have small, restless eyes set deep in the head. The principal symptom and the one that you must particularly remember, is that he will say he has always been near sighted. This information has led many an operator into prescribing minus lenses when the case was one of high degree hypermetropia. The fact that the retina is not well developed and his answers unsatisfactory regarding the test letters makes it all the easier to fall into this error. Do not be deceived, but determine once for all by a glance with the retinoscope just the true condition. The fact that he sees poorly at a distance and holds his book close in reading leads him to believe that he is myopic.

183. The name given to any uncomfortable feeling that is caused by eye strain.

184. As Examination No. 12 is a review I believe that a reference to some of the preceding lessons or rules will in many cases be productive of more good than a direct answer. In answer to this question I will therefore refer you to *Rules 12, 13 and 14*. The use of the visual angle is to enable us to determine size and distance.

185. *Rules 19 and 20.*   186. Any straight line drawn through the center of curvature except the one which strikes the mirror exactly in its center. The latter is called the principal axis.

187.–188. If the principal focus is at 10 inches (25 cm) then the object placed at 40 cm would come under *Rule 34*.   189. This would come under *Rule 36*.   190. See *Rule 35*. 191. At infinity.   192. Between the center of curvature and the principal focus, as close to the principal focus as possible, see *Rule 34*.   193. *Rule 36*. Close to the principal focus for the largest and close to the mirror for the smallest.   194. See Lesson No. 3, Fig. 13.   195. See the same diagram and *Rule 38*. The image will be larger than in the previous question. 196. See diagram 3 in Lesson No. 4 and the attending explanation.   197. See *Rules 39, 40, 41 and 43*.   198. The principal focus, in inches, of a plus 4 D lens is ten inches. One foot and eight inches is twenty inches. Hence we can find the answer in *Rules 46 and 49*.   199. See latter part of *Rule 50*. There will be no image. 25 cm is the principal focus of a 4 D lens.

200. Lesson 5, Fig. 5. Imagine the arrow IH to be the object and AB the image.   201. Hartridge, Fig. **43**. Imagine AB to be the arrow and the crystalline lens to be the convex lens.

202. Object at infinity. Image at the principal focus. *Rules 53 and 54.*   203. Against the lens.

204. 100 divided by 2.25 gives us practically 44 cm.

205. 100 divided by 40 gives us 2.50 D.   206. 40 inches divided by 8 gives us 5 D.
207. Minus 1.50 D.   208. I am sure that all of you can do this.

209. Superior, inferior, external, internal recti. Superior and inferior obliques.

210.–211. See answer to No. 101 in explanations on No. 5 and 6.

212. See *Rule 72.*   213. As the P. R. is at two meters we know him to be a myope of 0.50 D. An emmetrope would use 12.50 D of accommodation to see a 8 cm. The myope uses less than an emmetrope to the amount of his myopia. Therefore he will use 12 D to see at that point. Answer: 12 D.

214. An emmetrope would use 2.50 D to see at 40 cm. This eye has used 7 D to see at the same point. As he uses 4.50 D more than an emmetrope he must be a hypermetrope of 4.50 D and therefore his P. R. is 22 cm. behind his eye. (100 divided by 4.50 gives us practically 22.)

215. See *Rules 83 and 84.*   216. The hypermetrope's focus is behind the retina. When he looks across the street, or any other distance, he must accommodate and pull the focus to the retina or vision will be indistinct. We have learned that it is natural for convergence to act whenever accommodation acts and beyond certain limits the two are bound to act together. Therefore when the cilliary muscle exerts itself to bring the focus forward, the internal recti out of sympathy, also exert themselves although it is not desired. In other words the cilliary muscles act that the patient may see and the internal recti act just because they will not remain quiet when the cilliary are at work. The answer is not because accommodation and convergence are not in harmony, but because they ARE in harmony and are bound to work together.

217. 3 M. A. of convergence and 0.50 D of accommodation.

218.–219. See explanations on questions 90 and 91. Chromatic aberration may be overcome by making a convex lens of crown glass and a concave lens of flint glass in the right proportions and placing one against the other. Flint glass has greater dispersive power than crown, so it is not necessary to have the concave lens so strong as the convex in order for the aberration to be neutralized. The surplus of plus power in the combination is therefore the refractive strength of the "achromatic" lens.

220. In other words this 1.50 D hypermetrope puts a minus 3 D lens before his eye in order to see the patient's retina distinctly. Now a minus 3 D placed before a 1.50 D hypermetrope pushes the focus farther back and makes him a 4.50 D hypermetrope. In order to see he must therefore have converging rays to the amount of 4.50 D, for the hypermetrope is adapted to converging rays. Now the only eye that gives out converging rays is a myope. Hence the patient must be a myope of 4.50 D. In other words one defect just neutralizes the other. Hence the correcting glass is minus 3 D.

221. In this case the 1 D myope places a plus 3 D lens before him, thus making himself myopic 4 D in order to see the patient's retina distinctly. Hence the patient must be a hypermetrope of 4 D and the correcting glass is plus 4 D.

222. 2.50 D. See *Rule 101.*   223. A type of myopia which is progressive, becoming higher

in degree from year to year.　224. Usually by the pressure of the recti muscles on the sides of the long eyeball owing to the excessive convergence necessary in looking at near objects. 225. Optically the treatment consists in prescribing as near the full correction as can be used with comfort, together with grab glasses containing the remainder of the correction to be used as a convenience. Prisms, bases in, are a relief in many cases when reading as they lessen the convergence. The patient should avoid near work almost entirely, should have a good deal of out of door exercise and should form the habit of throwing the shoulders well back at all times to allow free circulation. However if there is a good oculist within reach he should be recommended.

226. Minus 10 for distance and minus 8 for reading, as explained in Lesson No. 12, beginning in the middle of page 2 and ending at the middle of page 3. Or, we could give him minus 10 for distance and tell him not to read for a week or two. By that time the accommodation would have become accustomed to working for it would be called upon each time that he looked at an object less than 20 feet away. Or, he could wear the minus 10 D for distance and take off his glasses for reading, as he has always done, for a week or two, and then gradually begin using the glasses for reading also. In short time he will leave them on constantly.

LESSON NO. 13.

Astigmatism.

HERETOFORE WE HAVE considered the lens and cornea as having perfect spherical surfaces, thus bringing rays to a focus at some point behind the lens. In this lesson we will consider a condition in which one of these media (usually the cornea) is not a section of a sphere, but is of shorter curvature in some of its parts than in others. The effect of such a refracting surface would be to bring rays, not to a focal point, but some of them would meet sooner than others, so that no matter where the retina might be placed it would be impossible to get all the rays together at the macula. This is known as "Astigmatism," Copy: *ASTIGMATISM.*

113. *Astigmatism is that condition of an eye in which the cornea (or sometimes the lens) has not the same radius of curvature for all its parts.*

114. *An imaginary line drawn across the cornea in any direction through its center is called a meridian.*

115. *Astigmatism is divided into two classes, Irregular and Regular.*

116. *Irregular Astigmatism is that in which the refraction differs in different parts of the same meridian.*

117. *Regular Astigmatism is that in which the refraction of one meridian differs from another, the meridian of greater curvature being at right angles to that of least curvature.*

Irregular Astigmatism may be caused by corneal ulcers; conical cornea (a disease in which the cornea protrudes forward); changes taking place in the lens, as in cataract; or by injury or operation on the cornea. A wound of any kind upon the cornea, would in healing be likely to draw or pucker the parts, forming something like a scar which would of course interfere with perfect refraction. All these conditions come under the head of Irregular Astigmatism. Very little benefit can be derived from glasses as it is impossible to grind lenses which will neutralize these irregularities. The cornea in its effect upon light, when in this condition, is very similar to a cheap mirror, that is, everything looked at has a "wavy" appearance. Stenopic spectacles sometimes aid in sharpening vision to a considerable extent. These consist of lenses ground partially opaque, simply letting light pass it at such places as the cornea is symmetrical in curvature, and shutting off rays that would strike the cornea at its irregular portions. These cases however should be referred to an oculist as they come more directly under his practice.

Regular Astigmatism is by far the most common form. This condition can be easily corrected by lenses and is one of the most satisfactory as well as profitable anomalies with which the optician has to deal. While the shape of the non-astigmatic cornea may be compared to the surface of an orange or ball, the curvature being equal in every meridian, the astigmatic cornea has a surface similar to that presented by the edges of a door-knob or a turnip. If you will consider such a surface for a moment you will see that it consists of two different curves, one a long sweeping curve, the other a short sharp curve, at right angles to the first. This is precisely the same condition that is found in the astigmatic cornea. Copy:

118. *The meridian of greatest curvature, and that of least curvature are known as the two "Principal" or "Chief" Meridians.*

119. *In the majority of cases the meridian of strongest (shortest) curvature is vertical, that of weakest curvature being horizontal. This is called "Astigmatism According to the Rule."*

120. *If the meridian of strongest curvature is horizontal, and that of weakest curvature vertical, it is called "Astigmatism Contrary to the Rule."*

121. *If the two principal meridians are neither vertical nor horizontal, but stand in an oblique direction, it is called "Oblique Astigmatism."*

There being two curves of different refractive power in the cornea rays passing through the meridian of greatest curvature must come to a focus sooner than those which pass through the opposite meridian. The retina interrupting these rays will receive images of different forms according to the distance at which it is placed from the lens. Hartridge, Figs. 76 & 77, shows these different forms very accurately, the rays VV representing those entering the vertical meridian, HH representing those in the horizontal. The vertical being the strongest meridian, these rays will come to a focus much sooner than the horizontal ones. If the retina is situated at 1 a large oval of diffused light is formed. If at 2, which is the focus for the vertical meridian, a horizontal line is formed, the vertical rays having met and the horizontal still on their way to a point. At 3 another oval of diffusion is formed, at 4 a circle of diffusion, the now diverging vertical rays crossing the converging horizontal rays at this point; at 5 an oval in the opposite direction appears; and at 6, the focus for the horizontal meridian we get a vertical line. Beyond this point we get a constantly increasing oval, always vertical, for the rays in the vertical meridian having crossed first have spread wider apart than those in the horizontal meridian.

If you will draw a cross upon the wall, and to each of the four ends tack the end of a string, you can easily demonstrate the formation of these lines and ovals. By drawing another cross on a piece of card board or cigar box, you can attach the other ends of the strings in such a way that they will represent rays entering and approaching the retina of an astigmatic eye. The string tacked to the upper end of the first cross should be attached to the lower end of the second, and that at the lower end of the first to the upper end of the second. The two strings from the right and left ends of the first cross should both be fastened together at the point of intersection of the second cross, that is, at the point where the two marks cross each other. Now draw them up tight and the wall will represent the cornea, the strings the rays, and the card board the retina. You will see that the vertical rays have come to a focus and crossed before reaching the retina, while the horizontal rays have just met at the retina. If you will hold the string still in this position and imagine the retina to be placed in each of the positions shown in the diagram referred to, I think you will clearly understand how the lines and ovals come to be formed. For instance, at the focus of the vertical rays a horizontal line is formed, at the focus of the horizontal rays a vertical line. At one point between the two foci where the converging and diverging rays intersect is a perfect circle. This point is called the "Focal Interval." At all the other points are found ovals, some vertical, some horizontal, according to the situation of the point. Take plenty of time to this experiment and study it carefully. It will be of more value to you than hours of reading on the subject.

The Astigmatic eye having two foci, one for rays entering the meridian of greatest curvature and the other for rays entering the meridian of least curvature, we may divide regular astigmatism into five classes according to the relative position of these foci to the retina. Copy:

122. Regular Astigmatism is divided into five classes according to the relative position of the foci to the retina.

123. One focus upon the retina and the other back of it, is called Simple Hypermetropic Astigmatism. (*See* Hartridge Fig. 79.)

124. Both foci back of the retina, one a greater distance than the other, is called Compound Hypermetropic Astigmatism. (*See* Hartridge Fig. 80.)

125. One focus upon and the other in front of the retina, is called Simple Myopic Astigmatism. (*See* Hartridge Fig. 81.)

126. Both foci in front of the retina, one a greater distance than the other, is called Compound Myopic Astigmatism. (*See* Hartridge Fig. 82.)

127. One focus in front and the other back of the retina, is called Mixed Astigmatism. (*See* Hartridge Fig. 83.)

The causes and symptoms of Astigmatism being thoroughly covered by Hartridge, a repetition will be unnecessary. The most frequent complaint is headache. Let us now consider the lenses used in correcting this defect and the manner in which they are placed. We will take for example a case of simple myopic astigmatism, Hartridge Fig. 81, in which one meridian is emmetropic, the other myopic. We will suppose the horizontal to be the emmetropic meridian, and the vertical to be myopic 1 D. How will we place this myopic focus back to the retina without disturbing the other focus which is already correct? If the case was one of simple myopia we could easily move the focus back with a concave spherical lens of the right power, but such a lens effects every meridian alike so that while we might be able to move the myopic focus back to the retina the emmetropic focus would move behind the retina, leaving us no better off than before. We must have a lens then which will be capable of refracting rays in one meridian, the meridian at right angles not being effected. The cylindrical lenses found in every good trial case are constructed upon this principle. These lenses instead of being segments of spheres, are segments of cylinders, being curved in one direction but straight in the other. A tin can or a lead pencil presents such a surface. If you will look lengthways along them you will see that they are perfectly straight but a glance across them shows a convex surface. This is the surface of a convex cylindrical lens. Now if you will look inside the can you will see a concave cylindrical surface. It is easy to understand that rays passing though a cylindrical lens in one meridian will be refracted while those in the meridian at right angles will not be refracted in the least. This last meridian is called the axis of the cylinder. Copy:

128. Regular Astigmatism is corrected by means of cylindrical lenses.

129. A cylindrical lens is one whose surface represents a segment of a cylinder, a curve in one direction, and a plane surface in a direction at right angles to the curve.

130. That meridian of a cylindrical lens which is a plane surface is called "The

Axis" of the lens, and rays passing through this axis will undergo no refraction.

In the case under consideration, simple myopic astigmatism 1 D, we have the horizontal meridian emmetropic, the vertical myopic 1 D. If we place a − 1 D cyl. before this eye with the axis horizontal, the horizontal meridian will remain unchanged while the vertical meridian will be corrected, thus moving the focus back to the retina. The eye will then be in an emmetropic condition (the lens being on) for parallel rays entering it in any meridian will be focussed upon the retina. − 1.00 D cyl. ax., Horizontal is therefore the correcting glass for this eye.

Let us next consider a case of compound hypermetropic astigmatism as shown in Hartridge Fig. 80. We will suppose the vertical meridian to be hypermetropic 1 D and the horizontal meridian hypermetropic 2 D. In this case neither of the foci are upon the retina and we must devise some means of correcting not only one meridian but both. This can be done by the use of a spherical and cylindrical lens combined. That is, we must place both lenses before the eye in order to correct it. We will first place a plus 1.00 D sph. lens before the eye. This being a spherical lens will effect all meridians alike, bringing the first focus to the retina, and the second dioptre nearer than it originally was. This will leave us with the vertical meridian emmetropic and the horizontal meridian 1 D hypermetropic. To bring this last focus up to the retina we must place before his eye plus 1.00 D cyl. ax. vertical. This will correct the horizontal meridian but will have no effect upon the vertical. We have therefore corrected this case by the use of a plus 1.00 D sph. lens in combination with a plus 1.00 D cyl. lens axis vertical. Of course we cannot give the patient two lenses to wear before one eye, for that would hardly be practicable. We must therefore send an order to the factory for a lens so ground that it will have the same optical effect as the two lenses combined. In order to do this we must understand writing prescriptions, and a word of explanation on the subject of prescriptions would not be out of place here.

The trial frames which usually come with trial cases, consists of a pair of adjustable frames with grooves in which to set the lenses. Around these grooves on either eye, is a metal scale marked off in degrees. The vertical meridian is marked 90, the horizontal 180 or 0, so that we have a complete half-circle marked off in divisions of 5 each, from 0 at one end of the horizontal meridian, around to 90 on the vertical meridian, and so on to 180 at the opposite end of the horizontal meridian. Wherever the axis of the cylinder happens to be placed we have only to glance at the trial frame in order to write the exact position. Instead of saying that two lenses are to be combined we have the sign ⊃ which means "combined with."

With this understanding we can easily write a prescription for the case at hand, which will read as follows: plus 1.00 D sph. ⊃ plus 1.00 D cyl. ax. 90. This means that we wish a plus 1.00 D spherical lens combined with a plus 1.00 D cylindrical lens, the axis of the cyl. to at 90, or vertical. Let us again consider the same case and see if we cannot discover a still different method of correcting it. The plan which we followed was to first correct the vertical meridian by means of a spherical lens, afterwards correcting the horizontal meridian with a cylinder. This procedure can be reversed with equal accuracy. That is, we may correct the horizontal meridian with a sphere and the vertical with a cylinder. This is done by first placing a plus 2.00 sphere before the eye, which will place the second focus upon, and the first focus one dioptre in front of the retina, and in addition a − 1.00 D cyl. with its axis horizontal, which will throw the now myopic focus back to the retina without disturbing the one already corrected. We have therefore two combinations from which to choose and we may write the prescription in either of the following forms: plus 1.00 D sph. ⌒ plus 1.00 D cyl. ax. 90, or plus 2.00 D sph. ⌒ − 1.00 D cyl. ax. 180. Either of these prescriptions are perfectly accurate, and although composed of combinations entirely different from one another, we will find in the lesson on lenses that the optical effect is precisely the same in each.

We will next consider a case of mixed astigmatism Hartridge Fig. 83. Let us suppose the vertical meridian to be myopic 1 D, and the horizontal hypermetropic 1 D. We have three ways in which to correct this condition. First, with a plus 1.00 D sph. which will correct the horizontal meridian and make the vertical 1D more myopic, combined with a − 2.00 D cyl. axis horizontal, which will correct the vertical meridian, leaving the horizontal still corrected, (plus 1.00 D sph. ⌒ 2.00 D cyl. ax. 180); second, with a − 1.00 sph. which will correct the vertical meridian and move the horizontal focus farther back, combined with a plus 2.00 D cyl. axis vertical, to correct the horizontal without again disturbing the vertical, (− 1.00 D sph. ⌒ plus 2.00 D cyl. ax. 90); third, with a plus 1.00 cyl. ax. vertical which will simply correct the horizontal meridian without affecting the vertical, combined with a − 1.00 D cyl. axis horizontal, which will correct the vertical without affecting the horizontal, (plus 1.00 D cyl. ax. 90 ⌒ − 1.00 D cyl. ax. 180). The last prescription is given the name of "crossed cylinders." All three of these methods are perfectly correct, all in reality having the same optical effect.

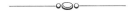

How may we test and measure astigmatism? Before answering this question, let us consider the action of an astigmatic eye. We will suppose for instance that the patient comes to us having compound Hypermetropic Astigmatism, the vertical meridian being 2 D hypermetropic and the horizontal 4 D hypermetropic. We seat him 6 meters from the test types and ask him to read aloud the smallest line of type he can make out. He reads say 6/18. This could not have been accomplished with the two foci behind the retina, so there must be some means in his power by which he can improve the condition. This is easily explained, for he has only to use 2D of accommodation in order to move the first focus up to the retina, the second moving forward 2 D. This is exactly the condition of his eye as he looks toward the test types.

Of course we are in ignorance of his true condition and have seated him in the chair for the sole purpose of finding it out. We therefore begin as usual with plus sphericals to see if vision still remains as good. In this present condition he certainly will see as well, for the plus lens only takes the place of his accommodation. For instance we place a plus 0.50 D before his eye and ask him if he sees just as good. He will answer that he does see just the same. We next place a plus 0.50 D over the first making a total of plus 1.00 D with which he still sees just as well, the only change going on in his eye being the relaxation of his accommodation. We still continue to increase the convex power, his accommodation steadily relaxing, until we have reached a total of 2.00 D when the accommodation is entirely relaxed. What will be the effect if we still increase the convex glass? Will he still see just as good or will the vision be worse? For instance let us add another plus 0.50. As his accommodation is now entirely relaxed, this lens will have the effect of bringing the first focus forward to a position in front of the retina, the second focus also moving forward but still remaining back of the retina. In this position he would certainly not see as well, for it is better to have even one focus upon the retina than neither. But the eye always makes an effort to see the best it can under all conditions and it has only to accommodate once more and bring the second focus to the retina (the first moving farther forward) in order to see equally as well as before. He therefore still accepts convex lenses and we may continue to add them until the accommodation has once more relaxed, at which time plus 4.00 D will be before him. We now have the eye perfectly quiet, for he cannot relax farther, and to accommodate again would make vision worse. We add another stronger lens but he sees worse, so we go back to the plus 4.00 knowing that at least one meridian of the eye is corrected and if there is astigmatism the uncorrected meridian now has its focus in front of the retina, in fact is myopic. The next question is to determine if he has astigmatism or if we have corrected a simple case of hypermetropia. If astigmatism is present, the now emmetropic meridian will certainly see better than the myopic meridian so we direct him to look at a chart similar to Fig. 84, Hartridge, and ask him if the spokes in the wheel look all alike, or if some are more distinct than others. If there is a difference we know that astigmatism exists, and next ask which spoke is the most distinct, in order than we may know which meridian is corrected. In the case under consideration he will say the vertical, and we then know that the horizontal meridian is the corrected one, for as explained by Hartridge we always see vertical lines with the horizontal meridian, horizontal lines with the vertical meridian of the eye.

The balance of the test simply consists of placing concave cylinders before the eye with their axis horizontal (for the horizontal meridian being already corrected we do not wish to again disturb it) until the vertical meridian is corrected, when the patient will tell us that the spokes all look alike, and the vision for the type will be at its best. When this is done we turn the cylinder slightly one way and the other, to make sure that we have placed it in just the right position, stopping when the patient sees best, and last of all we once more try plus sphericals to see if we cannot draw the accommodation out to a greater extent than before.

This can usually be done, for it is easy to understand that the cilliary muscle will hardly assume so complete a state of rest while embarrassed by astigmatism, as will be the case after the astigmatic condition has been corrected by cylinders. The other eye is now corrected by the same method after which both are uncovered and plus lenses once more tried, which ends the examination.

In compound myopic astigmatism (Hartridge Fig. 82) a convex lens would make vision worse by bringing both foci farther forward, so we must try concaves. These will make vision better step by step, until the posterior focus touches the retina when the patient will have as good vision as spherical lenses are capable of giving him. With any stronger minus lenses he will simply say he sees just as well, but not better, so of course we stop at the weakest, the same as in simple myopia. Next we ask him about the wheel and if some spokes are blacker than others we know that astigmatism exists, and also know that the uncorrected meridian is still in front of the retina. We must therefore use concave cylinders with the axis placed at right angles to the black spoke in order to move the uncorrected meridian back to the retina, when the astigmatism will be neutralized. We then slightly rotate the cylinder each way in order to get the best position, and end by trying plus lenses over the combination to see if the minus lenses already on, cannot be made a little weaker with equal satisfaction to the patient. If he accepts them we have induced the cilliary muscle to once more relax a little, which is always desirable.

Tests of all the different forms of regular astigmatism are made upon the same principle. We simply fit the eye in the same manner as we would simple hypermetropia or myopia, and after the strongest plus, or weakest minus lens is given, we know that at least one meridian is corrected and that if there is astigmatism the uncorrected meridian will, in the majority of cases, be now myopic. We have simply to place cylinders before the eye at right angles to the blackest spoke in the wheel, of the right strength to make the spokes alike, and after making sure of the correct position for the cylinder and trying plus lenses to relax as much accommodation as possible, we can rest assured that the eye is correctly fitted.

Some patients however will tell us that they see worse when the first focus is raised off the retina even though the second focus is still behind the retina. The reason for this is that they have not sufficient accommodation to bring the second focus forward, owing to its being too far back, or too weakened accommodation from old age. In these cases of course the minus cylinder will make the contrast between the spokes greater, and we will have to remove it and try plus in its place. In the majority of cases however the uncorrected meridian will be made myopic by the spherical lenses so that the chances will be in our favor of beginning with a minus cylinder. In those cases where it does not apply, it is an easy matter to lay it down and try a plus, always being particular to place the axis of either, just at right angles to the black spokes in the wheel. The following rules may be deducted for testing and fitting astigmatism. Copy:

> 131. *In correcting astigmatism subjectively, first make the usual tests for hypermetropia or myopia stopping with the strongest convex lens which maintains, or the weakest concave lens which gives, best vision. Next if there appears a difference in distinctness between different radiating lines, place cylindrical lenses (usually concaves) before the eye, with axis at right angles to the most distinct lines, until all radiating lines look alike. When this is done rotate the cylinder a few degrees each way to make certain of the correct position, and finish by trying once more to induce the patient to accept stronger convex sphericals.*

> 132. *In measuring an astigmatic eye by the Direct Method of Ophthalmoscopy, the observer finds the lens in his ophthalmoscope which gives a distinct view of the blood vessels running in one direction, and after making a note of this finds the lens which gives a distinct view of the vessels running at right angles to the first. The two lenses give the measure of the two meridians and a prescription can be written accordingly.*

> 133. *In determining the existence of astigmatism by the indirect Method of Ophthalmoscopy, the observer fixes his attention upon the optic disc and draws the strong convex lens toward him as usual. If the disc appears to change form, astigmatism is present. For instance if the height of the disc remains the same,*

the width increasing, or if the width remains the same the height increasing, we
have a case of Simple Myopic Astigmatism; if both height and width increase,
but one more rapidly than the other, it is Compound Myopic Astigmatism; if
height or width decreases the other remaining stationary, it is Simple
Hypermetropic Astigmatism; if both decrease, but one more rapidly than the
other, it is Compound Hypermetropic Astigmatism; and if one increases while
the other decreases the case is Mixed Astigmatism.

134. In determining astigmatism by the "Concave Mirror at a Distance," if the
vessels in one direction are seen, while those running at right angles are invisible,
the case is one of Simple Astigmatism either myopic or hypermetropic according
to the direction taken by the visible artery when the observer's head is moved. If the
vessels are seen in all meridians, but upon moving the head first from side to side
and afterward upward and downward they appear to move faster in one direction
then another the case is Compound Astigmatism, either myopic or hypermetropic
according to the direction of the movement. If in one meridian the arteries move
with the head, while the opposite meridian they move against the head, the case is
Mixed Astigmatism.

135. In correcting astigmatism by Retinoscopy, the plus 1.00 D lens being placed in
position, pass the light across the eye in one meridian adding convex or concave
sphericals until that meridian is corrected. Then pass the light across the eye in a
direction perpendicular to the corrected meridian and if a movement of the
shadow is shown place a cylinder (convex or concave as required) before the eye
with its axis on the already corrected meridian. Continue to increase the cylindrical
strength until there is no movement in that direction, when upon removing the
plus 1.00 D sphere, the remaining combination will be the correcting lenses. In
Oblique astigmatism the chief meridians may be easily found, for when the light
is passed across the face horizontally, the shadow will appear to move in an oblique
direction. In this case the light should be passed across the eye in that particular
direction instead of horizontally, afterwards correcting the meridian at right
angles to the first. A very close correction can be given by this method, it only
being necessary to make a few slight alterations in position and strength of sphere
and cylinder, by the subjective test, in order to obtain an accurate fit.

In many cases of astigmatism the patient gets better vision by holding the focal
interval upon the retina than in any other way, on account of diffused circles giving
more perfect form to the object than a line or oval. At such times the patient may say
that all radiating lines look alike, for one meridian is as imperfectly focussed as the
other. A little stronger convex lens than the patient likes to accept may be of service
in these cases by bringing the focal interval in front of the retina thus forcing him to
see better in one meridian than the other, and causing a difference in the appearance
of the lines. Other patients having always been accustomed to astigmatic vision will
declare that the lines all look alike from the simple fact that they never saw different.
With such patients we can only determine the presence of astigmatism (subjectively)
by means of the pin-hole test. If after doing our best with sphericals the pin-hole still
improves vision, we must either determine the astigmatism by some of the objective
methods or try cylinders of different strengths and in different positions with a view

to getting better vision for the test types. The objective method is, however, the most correct and scientific way. In connection with this lesson I would advise a re-study of Hartridge chapters 4 and 5, dwelling particularly upon those portions which relate to astigmatism.

Lesson No. 14 will close the present series of technical studies. With Lesson No. 15 we begin practical work, including arrangement of examination room, handling the trial case, transposing prescriptions, etc., ending the course with a study of prisms and muscular asthenopia. Although it is not absolutely required, I would suggest if you have not a trial case and outfit already, that you could derive considerable benefit from the remainder of the course by getting one now, and in fact beginning to do optical work in a small way. The study of the practical lessons in connection with the experience you would be getting in that way, would greatly enhance the value of the course. You are in position to handle the majority of cases even now, and by the time the course is completed you will have already become familiar with the work, and will feel better prepared for business from having had the experience. If I can aid you in the selection of a trial case or outfit, I will gladly do so at any time.

For your study between mails, take the ninth chapter of Hartridge.

(*End of Lesson No. 13.*)

EXAMINATION NO. 13.

227. What do you understand by "Astigmatism"?

228. Define Regular and Irregular Astigmatism.

229. Into how many classes is Regular Astigmatism divided? Define each.

230. How would you fit a case of Mixed Astigmatism?

231. Write two prescriptions for the correction of a case of Astigmatism, the vertical meridian being 3.50 D myopic, the horizontal 0.75 D myopic.

232. For a case in which the vertical meridian is 0.50 D myopic, the horizontal 3.50 D hypermetropic.

233. Write a third prescription for the same case.

234. Write a different prescription which will correct the same condition as the following: + 0.75 D sph ◝ − 1.50 D cyl ax 180°.

235. Is the following prescription for the correction of Astigmatism according to, or contrary to, the rule: − 0.75 D sph ◝ + 1.75 D cyl ax 180°.

236. How would you proceed in determining and correcting astigmatism?

237. What kind of Astigmatism will the following prescription correct? + 1.00 D sph ◝ − 0.75 D cyl ax 90°.

LESSON NO. 14.

Anisometropia.

ANISOMETROPIA IS THE name given to that condition in which the refraction of the two eyes differ. For instance one eye may be hypermetropic 1.00 D, the other hypermetropic 1.25 D; one may be emmetropic the other hypermetropic or myopic; one may be myopic 1.00 D the other 2.00 D; one myopic, the other hypermetropic; one astigmatic the other not; both astigmatic but one in a greater degree than the other; in fact, any refractive difference in the two eyes constitutes a case of anisometropia.

Anisometropia, as stated by Hartridge, is divided into three classes: (1) "Cases where binocular vision is present"; that is, both eyes are used together in looking at an object. (2) "When the eyes are used alternately"; that is, only one eye is used at a time, sometimes one and sometimes the other, as for instance if one eye is emmetropic and the other myopic, the emmetropic eye will be used exclusively for distance and the myopic eye for reading. (3) "One eye is permanently excluded from vision," which usually occurs when the difference between the eyes is very great, for in that case the eye of greatest ametropia is so poor as to be practically useless in aiding the better eye.

Naturally we would say that the proper mode of treatment for such conditions would be a perfect correction of each eye separately, thus making each emmetropic and allowing them to work together in harmony. It certainly would appear so, but practice teaches us that but a small percentage of Anisometropes will accept or tolerate a full correction of each eye, especially if the refractive difference is very great. The reason for this is still a matter of discussion, no very satisfactory conclusions having been reached. Some authors claim that it is due to the different prismatic effects of the two lenses when looked through obliquely, others that the patient having always been accustomed to seeing under these conditions does not take kindly to the change but is perplexed and annoyed by the new state of things, while still others claim that one glass having a greater magnifying power than the other will give to one eye a larger retinal image than its fellow, thus making it impossible to fuse the two images into one. There are arguments for and against all of these theories, but whatever the cause, the fact still remains that the majority of anisometropes find it impossible to bear a full correction of their defect. We must therefore govern our treatment by the symptoms and circumstances attending each individual case. Some will bear a considerable difference between the two lenses, while others will not tolerate a quarter dioptre difference. Hence we can formulate no rules for the correction of Anisometropia but must content ourselves with giving each patient as near the full correction as he can comfortably wear, always giving the full correction to the best eye and letting the difference be made in the poorer eye. Sometimes it will be necessary to change the glasses once or twice after you had thought them to be correct, for the patient is likely to come back after a few days with complaints of asthenopia even when at first the glasses had seemed satisfactory. It is usually well to explain to the patient the nature of his defect so that he may not lose confidence in you providing the glasses are not quite right the first time. The following cases from my record book may be of benefit to you in studying the different phases of Anisometropia:

Mrs. F. age 57, R. E. hypermetropic 2.50 D, L. E. hypermetropic 4.00 D, with both eyes uncovered sees easier with a plus 3.50 D before the left eye than with full correction. Gave her R. E. 2.50 D, L. E. plus 3.50 D which she has worn constantly ever since (two and one-half years) with perfect comfort.

Boy age 8. Requires R. E. − 8.00 D. L. E. plus p.75 D sph. ⌒ − 2.00 D cyl. ax. 160. The left eye being the nearest emmetropic was given the full correction. With both eyes fully corrected and uncovered objects seemed to swim. With right lens reduced to − 6.00 D vision was a little better but still unsteady. By still reducing this lens a dioptre at a time while the boy continued to look toward the test types, vision was most satisfactory with − 2.00 D, I therefore prescribed R. E. − 2.00 sph. L. E. plus 0.75 D sph. ⌒ − 2.00 D cyl. ax. 160, which he has since worn with perfect comfort.

H. W. T. age 26. Requires R. E. plus 3.25 D sph. ⌒ − 0.50 D cyl. ax. 110 L. E. plus 3.75 D sph. Prescribed full correction which has given excellent satisfaction.

Mr. B. age 47. R. E. plus 2.75 D sph. L. E. plus 2.00 sph. Prescribed full correction which gives entire satisfaction.

Mrs. S. age 41. R. E. − 0.50 D sph. ⌒ plus 1.25 D cyl. ax. 85, L. E. − 6.50 D sph. ⌒ plus 1.25 cyl. ax. 95. With both eyes uncovered cannot tolerate the glasses a moment. By holding a plus 1.00 sph. before the left eye, thus reducing the − 6.50 D to 5.50 D vision is slightly improved but still far from comfortable. By continuing to reduce the left lens she finally decides in favor of − 2.25 before that eye. The following was therefore prescribed: R. E. − 0.50 D sph. ⌒ plus 1.25 D cyl. ax. 85. L. E. − 2.25 D sph. ⌒ plus 1.25 D cyl. ax. 95. She returned in a few weeks to say that she had tried the glasses faithfully but had been unable to wear them for any length of time as they proved tiresome, and she feared the difference in the two lenses was still too great. I then changed the left lens to − 0.50 sph. ⌒ plus 1.25 cyl. ax. 95 which gave her the same power in each eye, and which she has worn comfortably ever since.

M. M. M. Book-keeper, age 37, complains of chronic sick headache, from which he has not been free for two consecutive days for over 16 years. Has tried every headache remedy in the market and spent a great many dollars with physicians without relief. Does not think it can be caused from his eyes but comes to have them examined as a last resort. R. E. plus 0.50 sph. ⌒ − 0.75 cyl. ax. 170, L. E. − 0.75 cyl. ax. 170. V without glasses 6/12, with glasses 6/5. Prescribed full correction to be worn constantly. After two weeks he returned to say he had not had a single headache since using the glasses. That he had even tried to bring on one by going to a ball game one raw afternoon and standing bare-headed for a good portion of the time. To say that he was delighted would be but a mild statement. I saw him 3 months later and at that time he had not had a single return of headache, was feeling better than he had felt before for several years, and had gained 12 lbs. in flesh.

Although we can lay down no iron-clad rules for the treatment of Anisometropia, the following are good general rules which I have used in my practice, always making such allowances however, as my judgment and the circumstances of the case led me to do. Copy: "*ANISOMETROPIA.*"

136. *Anisometropia is that condition in which the refraction of the two eyes are unequal.*

137. *In the treatment of Anisometropia always endeavor to give as near the full correction as the patient can wear with perfect comfort.*

138. *1.50 D is usually as great a difference as any patient will be able to bear and even that amount will be the exception rather than the rule.*

139. *Always give the best eye full correction, making the necessary alterations in the poorer eye.*

140. *In cases of Anisometropia with Astigmatism it is usually safe to give the full correction of cylinders, making the necessary alterations in the spheres; provided of course that the cylindrical difference is not too great. Before prescribing for such cases however it is always necessary to so transpose the prescriptions that each cylinder has the same sign, that is, both plus or both minus.*

141. *In high degrees of Anisometropia where the eye of greater ametropia has very inferior visual acuteness, it is usually more satisfactory to give each eye the same strength glass.*

142. *In low and medium degrees where visual acuteness of both eyes (when corrected) is about equal, the patient will usually bear a considerable if not full correction of the anisometropia, especially if he is under 30 years of age.*

143. *In people beyond middle life who have never been accustomed to a correction of their Anisometropia, an effort to correct over 0.50 D to 0.75 D of difference is usually unavailing.*

Presbyopia.

We have already seen that from the age of ten years the power of accommodation gradually diminishes until at about 75 years it is entirely lost. Whenever this diminution of power has become sufficient to render reading (or work at the average reading distance) uncomfortable, the patient is said to have become "Presbyopic," and must resort to artificial aid in order to see distinctly near at hand.

Donder's Chart, as reproduced by Hartridge Fig. 89, shows the usual amount of accommodative power present in the eye at different ages. Although all people do not have exactly the same amplitude of accommodation at any given age, still there is much less variation than one would naturally suppose, so little in fact that we may safely rely upon this chart in at least ninety percent of our cases. Let us consider the chart, that it may be thoroughly understood. The row of figures across the top represents the age of the patient; the first row at the left gives the punctum proximum in centimeters; and the second row represents accommodative power in dioptres. The white line running diagonally across the chart shows the near point, or punctum proximum, the horizontal white line showing the punctum remotum, which in this case is at 0, or Infinity, thus showing the patient under consideration to be emmetropic. To find the near point of an emmetropic child of 10 years of age we have only to look where the diagonal line crosses the ten year line which we find to be at 7 cm. 7 cm then, is his punctum proximum. His amplitude of accommodation (the difference between the refractive power representing his far point and that representing his near point) is 14 D (14 D − 0 equals 14 D). At the age of 15 the lines cross at 12 D thus showing 12 D of accommodation with the near point at 8 cm. At 20 years the near point has receded to 10 cm and the accommodation diminished to 10 D. At 25 he has but 8.50 D of accommodation; at 30 he has 7 D; at 35, 5.50; at 40, 4; at 45, 3; at 50, 2, with the punctum proximum 50 cm away. At 55 we notice that the punctum remotum is also beginning to recede to the minus or negative side of the line, in other words "beyond infinity," thus showing that our emmetrope is becoming hypermetropic. This is not due to presbyopia or to the loss of accommodation for the punctum remotum represents the adjustment of the eye AT REST and is of course not influenced by the changes which are weakening its working power, but is caused by the crystalline lens becoming flattened by age and thereby losing a portion of its positive refraction. At this age then the patient has become hypermetropic 0.25 D, and as the punctum proximum is still on the positive side of infinity, his amplitude of accommodation is about 1.50 D (the difference between the two white lines). At 60 he is 0.50 D hypermetropic with 1 D of accommodation; at 65, 0.75 hypermetropic, with 0.75 of accommodation (just enough to overcome his hypermetropia and still see distinctly at infinity); at 70, 1.25 hypermetropic with 0.50 of accommodation (the punctum proximum is now on the negative side also, leaving 0.75 D of his hypermetropia absolute); at 75 he is hypermetropic 1.50 D with practically no accommodation; and beyond that age his "acquired" hypermetropia gradually increases, his accommodative power remaining entirely lost.

If we wish to consider an ametropic eye we have only to imagine the two left hand columns to be moveable and place (in our minds) the figures representing the punctum remotum of the patient, opposite the punctum remotum line. For instance if we are considering a myope of 1 D we will pull the columns down until the figures 100 and 1 stand opposite the horizontal line R. His punctum remotum is then at 100 cm, or 1 meter, his punctum proximum at six and two-thirds centimeters at the age of 10. The number of squares between the two lines still represents the amplitude of accommodation, and as in the case of the emmetrope, we find it at 10 years 14 D, at 15 years, 13 and so on, the only difference being in the situation of the near points. At the age of 55 we find the myopia beginning to lessen, at 67 it has disappeared leaving him emmetropic, and at 80 he has become hypermetropic 1 D. To consider a hypermetrope of 1 D we will push the columns of figures upward until the − 1 is opposite the horizontal line. At the age of 10 his punctum proximum is at 7.5 cm., and his punctum remotum 1 D behind his eye. At 55 his hypermetropia begins to increase, at 67 it has reached 2 D, and at 80 years 3 D. Let us now consider presbyopia and its treatment.

So long as the individual is able to see comfortably at the reading distance, presbyopia has not commenced, but as his amplitude of accommodation grows less and less the time must come, unless he is myopic more than 3 D, when the punctum proximum will have receded so far from his eye that he is unable to read for any length of time. The first indications are that the type begins to blur and run together, especially in the evening, and he finds he must hold the paper farther from his eyes than formerly in order to read at all. If he still persists in trying to read under these conditions his eyes will water and become inflamed, and he will be compelled to stop every few moments to rest his overtaxed cilliary muscles before he can once more proceed. What other muscles in the human body would be so constantly persistent in forcing beyond their powers of endurance, or think that it could be done with safety to health, and yet we find nine people out of ten who insist that glasses should never be worn until the patient is absolutely compelled to put them on.

Let us suppose that a customer comes to us saying that he is 45 years of age and that he wishes to be fitted with a pair of glasses to read with. We first sit him down by the trial case and make the usual tests for ametropia. We find, let us say, that he is emmetropic in each eye. What will we give him for the reading glasses? By consulting the chart we find, unless he is an exception to the rule, that he has an amplitude of accommodation of 3 D. Now by using 3 D of accommodation we know that an emmetrope can see at 33 cm, and as 33 cm (13 inches) is the usual reading distance, we would at first thought wonder why he is not able to still read without glasses. We must remember however, that the chart gives the entire amplitude of accommodation, that is, the full effort that the eye is capable of putting forth when under test. No muscle can work continuously hour after hour to the full extent of its power. A man who, when put to the test could lift 600 lbs. could not continue to lift that amount for half a day at a time. A horse that can trot in 2:10 in a one mile race, could not keep up that speed for 60 or 100 miles, but perhaps if allowed to take a pace only half as great, thus keeping back a portion of his strength as a reserve, he might be able to keep it up for hours together. The cilliary muscles act upon the same principle. It has been found that the eye can usually keep up a constant accommodative effort of from two-thirds to three-fourths its entire power, without becoming fatigued, as it then has a reserve strength of one-third or one-fourth of its total power. This being the case our patient can only use continuously about 2 D of his accommodation, or two-third of the whole. As he wishes to read at 33 cm, which requires 3 D of accommodation, and as he is only capable of using 2 D comfortably, we must give him a pair of plus 1.00 D lenses, to make up the 3 D. If he had been a hypermetrope of 2 D we should have at first given him plus 2.00 D to correct his defect, thus making him emmetropic, after which the plus 1.00 D lens would have been added to supply the deficiency in his accommodation. His reading glasses would therefore be plus 3.00 D. Had he been myopic 1 D, no reading glasses would have been necessary, for after making him emmetropic with a − 1.00 D, and adding to this for his presbyopia a plus 1.00 D, the two lenses would just neutralize one another leaving them equal to no glasses at all. Again, we know that a myope of 1 D has his punctum remotum at 1 meter and only requires 2 D of accommodation to see at 33 cm, and as he can use 2 D of his accommodation comfortably, no reading glass is necessary for the patient. We can advise him to wear his distance glasses on the street, as he has been accustomed to do, and to remove them when he wishes to read.

Of course every patient does not have exactly 3 D of accommodation at 45, nor does every one read and write at 33 cm. These exceptions must be watched for and allowance made for them when found. It is usually my plan in working by this method to first give the patient such a glass as is called for by the above reasoning, and afterward vary the strength a little in each direction until the glass is found which gives good vision at the desired distance, and the patient to move a paper a little ways farther and nearer than that distance, thus giving him as much range and variation as possible.

Let us suppose the next patient to be 50 years of age and that he is hypermetropic 2.50 D. We first set him down at the case and make the regular test for distance leaving the plus 2.50 D lens before his eyes. Next we look at the chart to see how much accommodation he should have at that age, and find it to be 2 D. As he can only use about two-thirds of his accommodation continuously we can only depend upon 1.25 D of his accommodation and must add a plus 1.75 D lens to make a total of 3 D for reading at 33 cm. We will give this patient then plus 2.50 for distance and plus 4.25 for reading. A patient 55 years of age has 1.25 D of accommodation and can use about 0.75. To make a total of 3 D he must therefore be given a plus 2.25 in addition to the glass given for distance. At 60 he has a little less than 1 D and can use about 1.50 D so we must add plus 2.50 to his distance correction. At 65 he has from 0.50 to 0.75 and can use from 0.25 to 0.50 and we add plus 2.50 or 2.75. At 70 he may be able to use continuously 0.25 D accommodation or he may not, so the amount necessary to add will be plus 2.75 or plus 3.00. At 75 and upwards he has no accommodation, so that we must give him the entire strength necessary for reading, which on the above basis will be plus 3.00. We can therefore deduct the following rules which may be followed very closely in presbyopic cases. Copy: *PRESBYOPIA.*

144. Presbyopia is that condition due to the regular diminution of accommodation by age, in which the patient finds it difficult to read or perform work at short distance.

145. Donder's chart shows the usual amplitude of accommodation at different ages although there are occasional exceptions.

146. An eye can generally use two-thirds to three-fourths of its amplitude of accommodation without fatigue.

147. 33 cm (13 inches) is the average reading distance. An emmetrope must therefore use 3 D of accommodation when he reads.

148. Convex power must be added to the distance correction equal to the difference between two-thirds of the patient's amplitude of accommodation and the refractive power represented by the distance at which he is to work.

149. In fitting presbyopes the following is a good practical rule: First make the regular tests for ametropia and place the glasses which you would prescribe for distance, before the patient's eyes. Next ask his age, and for reading add to the glasses already on as follows: At 45 add plus 1.00; at 50, plus 1.75; at 55, plus 2.25 at 60, plus 2.50; at 65, plus 2.50 to plus 2.75; at 70, plus 2.75 to plus 3.00; at 75 and over plus 3.00. The strength should be varied a little each way, always noting the farthest and nearest points at which the reading type can be read, and stopping when the desired working distance is midway between these two points.

150. In prescribing the first pair of reading glasses a quarter or half dioptre less than indicated in Rule 149 will usually be preferable, as the patient having never been accustomed to glasses will not take kindly to the full strength.

151. In patients under 45, unless paresis of accommodation is present, the

correction of their ametropia alone will be sufficient for both far and near. Hence
people under 45 can use one pair of glasses for all purposes while people over
that age cannot.

You will notice that the above rules for the correction of presbyopia, differ very
materially from those given by Hartridge. His plan is to add plus 1.00 for each five
years up to 62 beginning with 45. While I requested you to study Hartridge's chapter
on Presbyopia, it was simply that you might compare the two methods for I do not
wish you to adopt his system by any means. Hartridge's work is a perfect text book
in ever respect save this, but the rule which he lays down for the correction and relief
of presbyopia is certainly founded upon an imperfect basis. For example let us take an
emmetrope of 60 years, who wishes to read at the average distance, 33 cm. According
to Hartridge's method this patient will require plus 4.00 as his reading glasses. But
what will be the result if plus 4.00 is given him? It will have exactly the same effect
so far as adjustment is concerned, as if an emmetrope should accommodate 4 D, or
in other words it will make the patient myopic 4 D with his farthest point of distinct
vision at 25 cm. He must therefore hold his paper 25 cm from his eyes, using 4 MA of
convergence, but no accommodation whatever, in order to read. This will be neither
satisfactory nor comfortable, for in the first place the patient desires to read at 33 cm,
which he certainly cannot do through plus 4.00 lenses, and further, he has nearly
1.00 D of accommodation at his disposal, 0.50 of which he can easily use continuously
and with less effort than would be required to hold his accommodation at rest while
so much convergence is at work. The plus 2.50 lenses which are recommended for this
age in Rule 149 will certainly be far more comfortable, as you can easily demonstrate
to your satisfaction by giving a 60 year patient a presbyopic correction of 4 D and
watching the result. He will without doubt bring them back the next day saying that
they did not fill the bill, but "tire and draw his eyes." Of course by "presbyopic correction" is meant a glass of certain strength added to the correcting distance-glass.
Thus if you wish to try the experiment upon a hypermetrope of 2 D you must give
him plus 6.00.

Some opticians instead of fitting presbyopic cases by the age of the patient, measure the amplitude of accommodation in each individual case. This is a practice which
cannot receive too high encouragement as it does away with all guess work and depends upon no chart. To find the amplitude of accommodation a number of good
instruments called "dynamometers" may be found upon the market. Hartridge Fig. 33
shows one of the most practical forms of this instrument, and one which you can easily
make for yourself. In the cut a narrow slit is shown which is used in measuring convergence. On the opposite side should be drilled a row of tiny holes close together.
The candle being lighted and the tape attached as described by Hartridge, the patient
is directed to fix his eyes upon the row of holes while you gradually draw it closer to
him. As soon as he is unable to distinguish one hole from another, but sees the entire
row as a line of light, you know that the punctum proximum has been reached, and the
distance of the punctum proximum from the eye will indicate the amplitude of accommodation. For instance if the punctum proximum is found to be at 25 cm we
know that he has 4 D of accommodation. If at 20 cm, he has 5 D, etc. Of course in
making this test the patient must either first be made emmetropic by the correction

of his ametropia, or else that defect must be figured in when computing the accommodation. For example if the patient is a hypermetrope of 3 D and we find his punctum proximum to be 2 cm from the eye we know him to have 8 D of accommodation. This as you doubtless remember, was thoroughly covered in that "entangling" Lesson No. 7. Should the accommodation be so low that the patient's punctum proximum is too far distant to enable him to distinguish the holes at all, he can be rendered temporarily myopic by a convex lens two or three diotropes and the punctum proximum found as before. The convex lenses must then of course be subtracted from the result. After determining the amplitude of accommodation, two-thirds of the whole should be subtracted from the lens representing the desired working distance (usually 3 D) and the remainder will give the presbyopic glass. This glass is added to the distance correction and the work is done. Copy:

> *152. To correct presbyopia by considering the amplitude of accommodation, subtract two-thirds of this amplitude of accommodation from the glass which represents the desired working distance. The remainder thus found is added to the distance correction.*

Let us suppose the desired working distance to be 33 cm, the amplitude of accommodation 1.50 D and the refraction of the eye 1 D myopic. Two-thirds of accommodation (1.00) subtracted from the glass representing 33 cm (3 D) leaves a remainder of 2 D. This added to the distance correction (− 1.00) leaves a total of plus 1.00 D (plus 2.00 and − 1.00 combined leaves an optical effect of plus 1.00) which is the glass we prescribe.

We naturally wonder why the relationship between accommodation and convergence is not disturbed by the presbyopic changes, for in reading the convergence always remains the same through life, while the amount of accommodation used gradually decreases, until finally none remains. The generally accepted explanation is that the same cilliary effort takes place at all ages, but that the lens having become less elastic does not respond so readily and a lower degree of accommodative power results. That is, a man of 60 makes the same muscular effort in accommodating 0.50 D that he used in accommodating 3 D at the age of 30. Hence accommodation and convergence still work in harmony, a proof of which is shown when we prescribe too strong lenses in presbyopia, in which case they invariably pain the eyes. Were net convergence considered this could not occur, for the stronger the lens used the less accommodation is brought into play and consequently less strain. The asthenopia must be due to the effort of holding accommodation in check while the convergence is at work.

As a great many of our presbyopic patients are also astigmatic it is necessary to add the presbyopic correction to a combination of lenses. To do this we simply add to the spherical lens leaving the cylinder as it was. For example if the patient requires plus 0.50 sph. ⊃ plus 0.25 cyl. ax. 90 for distance, and a presbyopic addition of plus 1.00, the prescription for reading would be plus 1.50 sph. ⊃ plus 0.25 cyl. ax. 90. If the distance correction is − 1.25 sph. ⊃ − 0.50 cyl. ax. 180 and the presbyopic addition plus 2.25, the prescription for reading would be plus 1.00 sph. ⊃ 0.50 cyl. ax. 180, etc.

It will be seen that hypermetropes become presbyopic earlier and myopes later than emmetropes, for the former must always use more accommodation and the latter less, in doing near work. Thus a hypermetrope of 1 D will find himself presbyopic at

40 while a myope of 1 D will read well without glasses until about 50 years of age. The correction of the hypermetrope's defect will, however, make him emmetropic and no other addition will be necessary until about the regular age, 45. The myope, if corrected, should also be able to read well with his — 1.00 until about that age when he can remove the glasses for reading. One more point and we will close this subject. Nearly all presbyopic patients inquire how long their glasses ought to last without changing. Of course you will answer them correctly from what has already been learned, in the young class of presbyopes, but if you do not take second thought you will be likely to make an error in answering older patients. According to Rule 149 the same addition is made from about 70 upwards, so that one is apt to tell the 70-year patient that his glasses will last the remainder of his life. But look out. The rule says that plus 3.00 is to be added to his distance correction, but you will remember that the eye constantly increases in its hypermetropic tendency year after year, so although the presbyopic addition remains the same, the glasses must nevertheless be changed from time to time. It is always well for the patients to call once a year, that their eyes may be looked after, and any necessary changes be made.

Paralysis and Spasm of Accommodation.

These conditions are so well covered by Hartridge that only a passing glance is necessary. Paralysis and paresis (partial paralysis) receive the same treatment as we have already explained in the case of myopes whose accommodative power is weak from disuse. That is we give the patient a correcting glass for distance and add to it as weak a convex glass as he can comfortably read with, gradually diminishing the convex power as the muscles become stronger, until he can read with his distance glass. This of course applies to younger people and should not be confounded with presbyopia.

Spasm of Accommodation we have already considered. A good idea in making the tests, in which we suspect spasm to exist, is to place before the patient stronger convex lenses than he actually requires, gradually reducing them by adding weak concaves, and stopping as soon as the concaves fail to make him read more letters on the cards. Many stubborn cases will yield by this method which can not be brought out in any other way save by the use of atropine.

(*End of Lesson No. 14.*)

QUESTIONS ON LESSON NO. 14.

238. What would you prescribe for the following case who wishes glasses for both distance and near: R. V. 6/40. with — 7.50 D sph. V. 6/18. L. V. 6/9. With — 0.75 D sph. ⌒ — 0.50 cyl. ax. 180 V. 6/6. Age 53?

239. What would you give a 3 D myope 76 yrs. of age for distance, and what for reading?

240. What would you do for a patient, age 19 as follows: R. V. 6/8. With plus 0.50 D sph. ⌒ plus 0.50 D cyl. ax. 90 V. 6/5. L. V. 6/10 With plus 0.50 D sph. ⌒ plus 0.50 D cyl. ax. 90 V. 6/5. At reading distance can only read coarse print with the above glasses, but with plus 1.00 D sph. added can read the finest type. Careful examination shows no spasm of accommodation present?

241. What would you give this patient for distance: R. V. 6/9 With — 1.00 D sph ⌒ — 0.50 D cyl. ax. 90 V. 6/6 L. V. 6/30. With — 3.00 D sph. ⌒ — 0.75 cyl. ax. 75, V. 6/6.

242. If 60 yrs. of age what will you give him for reading?

243. What would be the reading glasses for a patient 48 yrs. old who requires for distance R. E. — 0.75 D, L. E. — 0.50?

244. For a patient 65 yrs. old who requires for distance R. E. — 4.50 L. E. — 4.75?

245. Tell me what you would do if a boy of 16 came to you complaining that his eyes pained him after reading a short time, and that he had to leave school on account of his eyes, but the test shows nothing wrong with vision, and he is to all appearance an emmetrope? Answer fully.

246. What would you give an emmetrope of 46 for reading who had never worn glasses?

247. What is the reading glass for a hypermetrope of 1.50 D whose amplitude of accommodation is 3 D?

248. Of a myope of 1 D whose amplitude of accommodation is 1.50 D?

EXPLANATIONS ON LESSONS NO. 13 AND NO. 14.

237. *Rule 113.* Or, that condition in which all the rays of light do not come to a focus at the same point in the eye.

228. *Rules 116 and 117.*

229. *Rules 122 to 127 inclusive.*

230. By using a plus sphere to bring the hypermetropic focus to the retina, and a — cylinder with axis at right angles to the black line to push the myopic focus back to the retina. We can also correct it with a — sphere and a plus cylinder, or with a plus cylinder and a — cylinder, but the first form is preferable.

131. First, a — 3.50 sphere to push the front focus to the retina, and a plus 2.75 cylinder with axis vertical to push the back focus forward to the retina from the place where the — sphere left it. Second: a — 0.75 sph. to correct the back focus and a — 2.75 cyl. ax. horizontal to push the front focus the remainder of the way, to the retina. Answer: — 3.50 sph. ⌒ plus 2.75 cyl. ax. 90, and — 0.75 sph ⌒ — 2.75 cyl. ax. 180.

232. — 0.50 sph. pushes the myopic focus to the retina and the hypermetropic focus 0.50 D farther back. Plus 4 D cyl. ax. vertical, brings the hypermetropic focus to the retina and leaves the other focus where it is. Or, plus 3.50 sph. corrects the hypermetropic focus and pushes the myopic focus 3.50 D farther forward. Plus 4 cyl. ax. horizontal brings the myopic focus to the retina without disturbing the other. Answer: — 0.50 sph. ⌒ plus 4 cyl. ax. 90, and plus 3.50 sph ⌒ — 4 cyl. ax. 180.

233. — 0.50 cyl. ax. horizontal corrects the myopic meridian without disturbing the hypermetropic. Plus 3.50 cyl. ax. vertical, corrects the hypermetropic meridian without disturbing the myopic. Answer: — 0.50 cyl. ax. 180 ⌒ plus 3.50 cyl. ax. 90.

234. The best way to solve this problem is to draw a diagram similar to those in Hartridge, page 162, and locate the two focal points. Then prove your diagram to be correct by seeing if the given prescription will correct the defect, and if so, write the second prescription for the same case just as I have done in the preceding question. Answer: — 0.75 sph. ⌒ plus 1.50 cyl. ax. 90.

235. In this case the horizontal meridian of the eye is the strongest. We know this be-

cause we placed a plus 1.75 D cylinder before the eye with its axis horizontal in order to make the vertical meridian as strong as the horizontal. It is therefore a case of astigmatism contrary to the rule. See *Rules 119 and 120*. If the vertical meridian were the strongest, it would be according to the rule.

236. This is quite fully explained in *Rule 131*. I cannot advise you too strongly to follow that rule in all cases. You will find it the quickest and most systematic way of fitting astigmatism that there is. Note particularly that the cylinders used in the test are nearly always minus; the reason for this is explained in Lesson 13. When the test is finished, you can transpose the prescription into any form you wish, but the minus cylinders are, almost without exception, the ones you will use during the test if you follow this system carefully.

237. Compound hypermetropic astigmatism, the horizontal focus 0.25 D behind the retina, and the vertical focus 1 D behind the retina; therefore, contrary to the rule. You can solve this problem in the same manner as suggested in No. 234.

238. For distance, RE − 1 D sphere, LE − 0.75 sph. ⌒ − 0.50 cyl. ax. 180. For reading, RE plus 1 D sph. LE plus 1.25 D sph. ⌒ − 0.50 cyl. ax. 180. (*Rules 141 and 149*).

239. − 3 D for distance corrects his myopia and makes him an emmetrope. This is the correct distance glass. For reading we add plus 3 D to his distance glasses (*Rule 149*) which is equal to nothing. Tell him to remove his glasses when reading.

240. The correcting distance glass as given. Also plus 1 D in grab frames to use in reading, gradually reducing them from time to time, as his accommodation becomes stronger. He ought to use his distance glasses for all purposes in a short time. The condition is paresis of accommodation.

241. The correction as given except that the sphere in the left lens should be made 2.50 D. (*Rule 138.*)

242. RE plus 1.50 D sph. ⌒ − 0.50 D cyl. ax. 90 LE − 0.75 cyl. ax. 75. (*Rule 149.*)

243. By adding plus 1.50 D to the distance glasses, for his age, we have RE plus 0.75 D LE plus 1 D. (*Rule 149.*)

244. In the same way we get the following: RE − 2 D LE − 2.25 D or RE − 1.75 D LE − 2 D. See *Rule 149.*

245. This boy is evidently suffering from one of two conditions. He is either an emmetrope as he appears to be and has weak accommodation (Paresis), or else he is a hypermetrope with a spasm of accommodation which just covers his defect. Atropine will tell us if the latter condition is his trouble, but if Paresis is the condition the use of Atropine would make a weak muscle weaker. However, in either case plus lenses would be the optical treatment. I would therefore suggest that we give him plus 0.25 D, for reading only, and have him use these glasses for a week or ten days and then come back for a second examination. By this time we can no doubt determine the true condition. If he is hypermetropic, some of the latent will have become manifest under the use of the glasses. In that case we can correct what we find and have him wear the glasses constantly instead of only for near work, following up the hypermetropia from time to time as more of it becomes manifest. If he is not hypermetropic, of course we will deal with him as in any case of paresis of accommodation.

246. The rule at the age of 45 is 1 D. This patient, being a year older, we would, according to *Rule 150*, give him about plus 1 D.

247. His total accommodation being **3 D,** he has only 2 D that he can use comfortably. The hypermetrope of 1.50 D uses 4.50 D in reading at **33** cm. As he can only accommodate comfortably 2 D we must help him the other 2.50 D with a plus lens. (*Rule 152.*)

248. A 1 D myope must accommodate 2 D in reading at **33** cm. This patient has 1.50 D of accommodation which means that he can use comfortably two-thirds of it which is 1 D, hence if he has 2 D of work to do, and can only do 1 D with comfort, we must help him with a plus 1 D lens. (*Rule 152.*)

L E S S O N   N O.   1 4. (Supplement.)

While Rule 149 is a good mathematical rule for the correction of Presbyopia still we cannot always follow mathematical rules in optics. The following rule based upon an extended experience in these cases, as well as in cases of paralysis of accommodation, which is really the same thing to a young person as Presbyopia is to an older one, will be of great service to you in prescribing reading glasses.

Rule: Correct the patient for distance and place before both eyes the lenses that you would prescribe for constant wear. Have him hold the reading types at the exact distance that he desires to work or read. Place before both eyes the lenses called for in Rule 149 according to his age. Over this hold minus 0.25 D, in each hand and ask the patient if he still sees just as well. If so reduce the presbyopic addition as far as he will accept. If minus is worse then take plus 0.25 in each hand and see if it decidedly improves vision. If so increase the presbyopic addition but only continue to increase it as long as it proves a decided improvement.

In other words add to the distance glasses the weakest convex lenses through which he can read best at the desired working distance.

You will find this rule almost infallible if applied in artificial light. In fitting the patient in daylight follow the rule in the same manner, but when all is finished prescribe plus 0.50 D more than found by the test. This will enable the patient to read in the evening as well as in the daytime.

With kindest regards I remain,

Yours Sincerely,

Dr. H. A. Thomson.

134

LESSON NO. 15.

Practical Work.

WITH THE EXCEPTION of Prisms and Muscular Anomalies which we will reserve until the last, we have now covered very carefully the technical portion of the course and are ready to begin practical work. The arrangement of a suitable room in which to make examinations is the first consideration.

It is essential that this room be as convenient as possible so that the necessary tests may be made quickly and systematically, without tiring the patient to an unnecessary degree. This may be done in a very simple and inexpensive manner. In nearly every store-room there is a space in the rear which can be utilized for this purpose. A room 7 or 8 feet wide, extending from the rear wall toward the front should be partitioned off, the inside measurement to be 21 feet in length. A doorway is cut in the front end, but no windows of any kind are desirable for we wish the room to be as dark as possible. At each end of the room a shelf or table should be built, one at the front for the trial case, the other for the reflector. I find the most convenient height for these shelves to be 26 inches for the front and 29 inches for the rear, measuring from top of the shelf to the floor. The front shelf should be about 16 inches in width by 52 inches in length, extending from the side wall toward the door. A notch or jog of sufficient size to admit the patient's chair is cut in this shelf. The rear shelf or table should measure about 29 inches in width by 52 inches in length, extending from the same wall.

The reflector consists of a sheet of tin 46 by 14, and should be rolled by the tinner so as to give it a curved surface, straight the long way and curved across, like a cylinder. The inner or concave surface should be given three or four coats of white paint, the back painted a dead black. Against the rear wall, a foot or so above the table, the test types should be hung. In my practice I use four of these cards. One German, two English, and the Astigmatism dial. The three long cards I place side by side, the middle one 6 or 8 inches higher than the other two and underneath the middle card I place the dial. I have never found it necessary to use any other cards than these, and too many are apt to be confusing. The reflector should be so placed upon the table that the lights will be reflected directly upon the cards, very much like the foot-lights in the theatre.

For illumination, either gas or kerosine may be used, or if there is a day circuit in your town, electric lights may be placed behind the reflector with the button at the other end of the room beside your trial case. The light used in ophthalmoscopy and retinoscopy however, should be gas or kerosine, as electric light is not so satisfactory for that purpose. If you use gas the following arrangement will be the most satisfactory. Have your plumber fit three ordinary burner tips, about 16 inches apart, into the side of a gas pipe, with a stop-cock at one end. Attach this to the main pipe where it comes up through the table, letting it lie in front of the reflector with the tips inclined toward it at an angle of about 45 degrees, so that when in use the light from the three burners will be thrown upon the wall. By this arrangement one stop-cock controls the three flames. In addition to these burners bring another branch of the main pipe up through the table on the opposite side of the reflector, that is, on the side toward the patient. To this pipe attach a complete burner with stop-cock, letting stand perpendicular just above the surface of the table. This burner is used for muscle tests and must work independently of the others. Against the wall at the upper end of the room some 20 or 24 inches above the shelf and directly over the right corner of the patient's chair, an oculist's adjustable lamp bracket, with Argand burner, should be screwed. These brackets can be procured of any wholesale optical house and are almost indispensable to the optician. If you desire to use kerosine instead of gas, two or three flat-bottomed lamps set in front of the reflector will answer every purpose. By turning down all but one, and setting that one on the other side of the reflector in view of the patient, the muscle test can be made. At the upper end of the room, the adjustable bracket with lamp holder may be used in the same manner as the Argand burner. In ordering a bracket state whether wanted for gas or oil, and the proper one will be sent you.

With a roomy arm-chair for the patient, a stool or chair for yourself and the trial case in position upon the shelf, the arrangement of the room is complete. The gas fixture, if your plumber is a man of taste, can be put in without exposing the pipe or interfering with the neat appearance of your room in any way. The finish of your walls may depend upon your choice. Although theoretically they should be painted a dead black to absorb superfluous rays, still the advantage derived will hardly compensate for the uninviting appearance of the room, pleasant tasteful surroundings often having considerable influence with customers, especially ladies. A good wall paper of not too light a shade will answer every purpose, and your work can be done just as correctly as would be the case were the walls black.

The above description is for an ideal room. The objective subjective and muscular tests may all be made while the patient sits comfortably in his chair, without confusion or loss of time. Of course if it is not convenient to do off a room in this manner, or if you contemplate making visits to other towns, different plans may be substituted with perfect satisfaction. Day-light, with the patient's back to the window, will suffice for illumination of the cards; a corner curtained off, with a stand and student's lamp within, answers every purpose in objective tests; and the same lamp placed 20 feet from the patient makes a perfect muscle test. Circumstances and surroundings will govern you in the matter of arrangement, the principal object being to make all the examinations as convenient as possible.

The amount of stock required also depends upon yourself. A great many only keep a very little stock on hand, as the majority of the work is done by prescriptions and the glasses made at the factory anyway. Some of my pupils commence with about $15.00 worth of stock and add to it as necessity demands. The following list covers a value of about $65.00 which is all that will be necessary in a good business, with the possible addition of gold frames from time to time. 4 medium weight 10K R. B. frames; 2 E. G. frames off-set guard 10K; 1 Skel E. G. off-set guard 10K with plus 0.50 lenses; 1 medium and one heavy 10K S. T. frames; 1 R. P. E. G. Chain, with hook; 1 R. P. hair-pin chain; 6 silk cords with hook and swivel; 3 silk cords without; 1 silk cord with

R. P. hook and swivel; 8 nickelled R. B. frames; 6 nickel E. G. frames off-set guards; 6 nickel E. G. frames plain guards; 12 nickel S. T. frames; 6 bronze S. T. frames; 1 gross cases with name on as follows: 2 doz. S. T. open end; 2 doz. S. T. closed end; 4 doz. R. B.; 1 doz. flat E. G. for plain guard; 3 doz. Patent off-set cases, and the following lenses: 2 pairs each convex by quarters 0.25 to 4.50, by halves 4.50 to 8.00. In concave, 1 pair each by quarters 0.25 to 3.00 and by halves 3.00 to 5.00 and one pair plano.

A \$15.00 stock would consist of the following: 12 nickel R. B. frames assorted; 12 nickel S. T. frames; 2 nickel E. G. frames off-set guards; 2 nickel E. G. frames plain guards; 1 nickel Skel E. G. off-set guard. Cases as follows: 6 R. B., 6 S. T. open end; 2 flat E. G. for plain guard; 3 Lloyd, not lettered. Lenses as follows: Convex 1 pair plus 0.25; 2 pairs each by quarters 0.50 to 3.75 inclusive; 1 pair each by quarters 4.00 to 5.00 inclusive; 1 pair each by halves 5.50 to 8.00, and 1 pair plano. No concaves. With this assortment a frame can be found of the proper dimensions to fit any face and a duplicate ordered of the material desired. The majority of your customers will require compound lenses which have to be ordered by prescription and it is as easy to order sphericals when necessary. Most people seem better satisfied if their glasses are "made for them" anyway, so there is but little disadvantage in carrying a small stock. Orders for convex sphericals in nickelled frames can of course be filled from your assortment.

With the examining room in order, and the goods received, you are now ready for customers. The following is, I believe, the best order in which to make the tests. First seat the patient in the chair and ask him in what way his eyes give him trouble. While listening to his history of the case make a careful scrutiny of his face and eyes, noticing the most prominent features. In this way you will be able to form an approximate idea of his condition before beginning the test. His description of the symptoms are also an important aid in diagnosing the case. Next ask him to look straight ahead toward the lower end of the room (which is still dark) and taking the ophthalmoscope in your hand make the "Concave Mirror at a Distance" test. This is quickly accomplished for you have only to move your head from side to side until you catch a glimpse of an artery and notice the direction it takes. One point regarding this test however, not mentioned in the books. That is, you must place a convex lens before the patient's eye to neutralize the distance of your eye from him. For instance if you are 50 cm from him a plus 2.00 will be required. This you can easily hold in your left hand while you hold the ophthalmoscope with your right. The next test should be the Direct Examination, which you make by taking away the convex lens and approaching the patient without once removing the ophthalmoscope from your eye. After making this test you can move back again to a distance of about twenty inches and taking a plus 13.00 from the trial case make the Indirect Examination, not forgetting to use the plus 2.50 lens in the ophthalmoscope. You can now lay away the ophthalmoscope, but before putting the plus 13.00 away, ask the patient to look directly toward you, while you examine his eye by "Focal Illumination," or, as it is sometimes called, "The Oblique Examination." This consists of throwing the light across the patient's cornea by means of a convex lens. Swing the lamp to the side, and a little forward of the patient's face so that the light will shine directly across his eye. Then hold the convex lens in such a manner that the rays passing through it will come to an intense focus at the cornea.

The cone of light thus passing across the cornea and iris will render it a very easy matter to detect and locate any opacities or ulcers that may be present on or underneath the cornea. With the exception of a preliminary examination with the retinoscope, which you may now make if considered necessary, the objective examinations are at an end, and you are ready to begin with the trial case. The foregoing examinations, although it has taken some little time to describe can be easily made in one or two minutes.

By this time a very good idea of the patient's condition has already been formed and the trial case examination may be very easily made. A few points regarding the correct method of handling the trial case with greatest comfort to the patient, would not be out of place here. Let us suppose our patient is a hypermetrope of 3 D, all of which is facultative. Of course we are not aware of his condition, but we proceed by the regular methods to ascertain it. Beginning with a plus 0.25 we hold it before the uncovered eye and ask him if he can see as well, which of course he can. Now at first thought we would be inclined to lay that glass down and take up the plus 0.50 asking him the same question, lay the 0.50 down and try plus 0.75, and so on until we found the strongest glass through which he could see just as good. But let us stop and consider the effect such a procedure will have upon the eye. First, as the patient looks toward the cards without a glass, he is using 3 D accommodation to bring the image upon the retina. When we place plus 0.25 before him, the accommodation relaxes 0.25 and the image still remains upon the retina. Now as we remove the glass he must once more accommodate 3 D. As he looks through the plus 0.50 he again relaxes, a little more this time and as we remove the lens he accommodates 3 D as before. The plus 0.75 causes a still greater relaxation and its removal another exertion, and so on, until by the time we have reached the full measure of his defect, the eyes are tired and irritated, and in the majority of cases a spasm of accommodation brought about, which will greatly interfere with the accuracy of the test. This is certainly an undesirable condition and should be avoided in every way possible. Tests made in this way by careless opticians are the cause of many people putting off and dreading an examination owing to the prevailing opinion that a test of the eyes is tiresome in the extreme and will usually cause a severe headache for hours afterward. Any optician who understands the mechanism of the eye, and has due regard for the patient's feelings, as well as his own success in making an accurate examination, can avoid this result by using ordinary care during the test.

Let us begin as before with plus 0.25 asking the patient if he can see just as well. As he says he can we leave the lens before his eyes in the trial frame, and taking up the other plus 0.25 hold it also before him, asking the same question. As he still sees as well we place this lens in the frame with the first, making a total of 0.50 D before his eye. The frame now being full and both 0.25 lenses in use, we must make some change in order to proceed with the test. We accordingly take a plus 0.50 in the right hand, holding that hand in such a manner that either the hand or coat-sleeve comes between the patient's eye and the test types, and withdraw the two lenses from the frame with the left hand, at the same time inserting the 0.50 in their place. We now have the same power before his eye as before, but once more have room in the frame for another lens and have the 0.25 lens in the case for further use. Placing one of these in the frame and asking the old question, we insert the 0.75 in the same manner as we did the 0.50. This is continued until the limit is reached when the examination of that eye will have been completed without a single effort on the part of the patient's eye. This method of building up lenses is an important point and should be followed in all cases.

In correcting hypermetropes whom we suspect of having spasm of accommodation, the following plan often enables us to draw out a part of the latent defect. Instead of beginning with the weak convex glass and gradually working up to the strongest he will accept, we begin by placing a convex glass before him, somewhat stronger than we suspect his hypermetropia to amount to. This of course overcorrects him and by bringing his focus too far forward, renders him artificially myopic. Of course he will not see well, but we proceed precisely as in myopia using weak concave lenses until he can see the same line he has previously read. The combination thus forms the measure of his manifest hypermetropia, usually more than would be shown by the ordinary method.

Another feature of the trial case examination regarding which we should be particular is the method of questioning the patient. For example, we will suppose him to be a young hypermetrope, and that upon asking him to read the test types his vision is 6/6. We of course begin by placing before him a weak plus glass and ask him a question. Now what shall that question be? Our first inclination would very likely be to ask: "Is this better?" But is that what we want to know? Do we not know before he tells us, that it will not improve vision in the least, for his accommodation had already brought the image to the retina before we used the lens, so that the only change that took place in his eye, was the relaxation of the cilliary muscle. This will certainly not improve his vision, or even change it, so that it would certainly be absurd to ask him if he saw better. Our aim in fitting him is to find the lens that makes him see WORSE, for when that lens is found we know that the one tried just previous to it is the measure of his hypermetropia. It would be much more to the point to ask him if he "sees worse" than to ask if he "sees better." "Can you read the same line through this"; "Is this just as good"; "is this just as good or worse"; etc., are the correct questions in applying convex lenses. Of course there are cases where a part of the hypermetropia is absolute, in which the convex lens improves vision by accomplishing what the cilliary muscle was unable to do, but even then it is not necessary that we ask if he sees better, for so long as he even sees "as well" we will continue to add the lenses. If he does see better he will very likely tell us so, but the only part that interests us is to find a glass just strong enough to make him see worse again, so that the same question should be asked in every case. Begin a new page in your note-book, heading it "*PRACTICAL HINTS*," and Copy:

153. Never, under any circumstances, ask the patient if he can see "better" while applying a convex glass. Simply ask if he sees "just as well."

In correcting myopia, and using concave lenses, the case is different. In the myope the image is in front of the retina, thus rendering the vision imperfect. Each minus lens that we place before him carries the image farther back, and we naturally expect him to see better. In fact we must refuse to give him the glass unless he does. We will take for illustration a myope of 1 D. The − 0.25 makes him see better by bringing the image closer to the retina. So likewise, do the 0.50, 0.75 and 1.00. But as the − 1.00 brought the image upon the retina, making him practically an emmetrope, he is now seeing at his best. The next lens, − 1.25, carries the focus still farther back, making him hypermetropic, which he at once corrects by bringing it back again with the power of his accommodation. He still sees "just as well" but of course no better, and we certainly do not wish to over-correct him in this manner, and leave him to accommodate for all distances. Hence we take the last lens off again and prescribe the − 1.00. So we must never prescribe a concave lens unless the patient declares, and proves by his reading, that he sees better. Our question then in applying concave lenses will be: "Can you see better?" Copy:

154. In applying concave lenses always ask the patient if he can see "better," and do not prescribe a concave lens under circumstance, if he only sees "just as well" and not "better."

As the lesson so far has covered nothing which requires study, we will now postpone the practical talk until next time, and devote the balance of our space to the consideration of a few problems in prescriptions. When we correct a case of astigmatism in which both a spherical and cylindrical lens have been used, for example, a plus 0.50 spherical and a plus 0.75 cyl. with its axis vertical, we write a prescription like this: plus 0.50 sph. ⊃ plus 0.75 cyl. ax. 90. Up to this point the subject has already been covered in the preceding lessons, but the refractive strength of the lenses considered in their combination, have never been discussed. If two spherical lenses, as − 1.00 and − 0.50 are placed in combination, we know at once that the result is − 1.50, but when spherical and cylindrical lenses are combined, the problem is not so readily solved. Let us take the above prescription as an illustration and analyze its powers. The first lens in this prescription is plus 0.50. This lens when placed in the trial frame alone, has a refractive power of one-half dioptre in the vertical, horizontal, and in fact every meridian. Now let us place the plus 0.75 cyl. also in the frame with its axis at 90. The axis of a cylinder as we know, has no effect upon rays of light, being perfectly straight like a plane glass, hence in the vertical meridian the original power has not been effected in the least, still remaining 0.50. In the horizontal meridian however a marked change has taken place, for a cylinder in the meridian at right angles to its axis has all the power of a spherical lens. In this meridian therefore, we have power equal to the two lenses combined, (plus 0.50 and plus 0.75 makes plus 1.25). Our combination then, has refractive power of plus 0.50 in the vertical meridian and plus 1.25 in the horizontal which we may express by a cross as shown in the diagram.

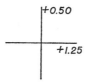

The examination in this lesson consists of a number of prescriptions from which you are to draw similar crosses. This is a beginning of the series of exercises in the study of combinations which we will continue through the next two or three lessons.

QUESTIONS ON LESSON NO. 15.

Make a cross showing the power in both vertical and horizontal meridians in the following combinations.

249. plus 1   ◡   — 1.50 ax. 180.
250. plus 3.75 ◡ plus 1.   ax. 90.
251. — 0.75 ◡ plus 3.   ax. 90.
252. — 4.   ◡ plus 3.   ax. 180.
253. plus 3.   ◠ — 3.   ax. 180.
254. — 1.50 ◡ — 3.75 ax. 90.
255. plus 7.   ◠ — 6.   ax. 180.
256. plus 3.   ◠ — 8.   ax. 90.
257. plus 4.   ◡ plus 9.   ax. 180.
258. — 1.   cyl. ax. 90.
259. plus 3.   cyl. ax. 90.
260. — 6.   ◡ plus 6.   ax. 180.
261. — 3.   ◠ — 4.   ax. 180.
262. — 4.   ◠ — 4.   ax. 90.
263. plus 4.   ◡ plus 4.   ax. 180.

LESSON NO. 16.

Practical Work. (Continued.)

IN TESTING AND fitting hypermetropia we have always said that the strongest convex lens through which the patient can see as well is the mesure of the defect, and we have even gone so far as to leave the glass before the eye if the patient could still make out the same line as before. Now while this is all right in principle, still I wish to caution you against being too iron-clad in following rules. It is sometimes a question whether the last quarter will be as acceptable to the patient, when he comes to wear the glass as without it. An over-correction, of course makes the patient myopic, which blurs vision for distance and naturally causes dissatisfaction. I notice the tendency with pupils is to give the very last glass up to the limit of seeing worse, which is in accordance with their instruction, but will result in the glasses very frequently being too strong. In my practice I usually make it a rule to gradually increase the convex power until the vision is decidedly worse, when the glass that rendered it so is of course removed. This leaves us at the limit glass and the question is, shall we prescribe this or make it a quarter weaker. Of course if the patient is showing symptoms of spasm of accommodation then I will give the full correction, for it is desirous that the spasm be drawn out to its fullest extent, but in the ordinary types of hypermetropia I find it does no harm to allow the patient to choose for himself between the two. This may be accomplished by leaving the full correction in the frame and holding the weakest concave lens, one in each hand, before him, and alternately removing and replacing them until he is positive which one he prefers. If there is no preference whatever, then give him the strongest, but in young hypermetropes with strong accommodation it usually gives better satisfaction if they are allowed to give their accommodation a little surplus range. Do not over-do this matter and prescribe too weak lenses, but what I wish to impress is that we are to use practical common sense in our work, and not be guided entirely by absolute rules.

The same principle holds good in the use of concave lenses except that the question is reversed. "Shall we give the very weakest glass through which the patient can possibly distinguish his best line, or shall we make it an eighth or a quarter stronger?" He may also be given his choice in this matter, but his choice must have the support of your judgment which is based upon his answers. If he really sees the line better and can read it more readily, then you will be safe in giving the stronger lens, but if he only says that the letters look blacker, but does not read them any more readily than before, it is better to give the weaker glass, for concave lenses always have the effect of condensing and blackening the letters.

Having passed through the preliminary stage, and placed before the eye the proper spherical lens, we next direct our attention to the examination for astigmatism. It is at this point that many students in optics come to a standstill, seeming to feel that they have reached the foot of an unsurmountable hill. How often one hears the following remark: "I can fit ordinary cases, like hypermetropia, myopia or presbyopia, but when it comes to astigmatism it is altogether too complicated for me to handle." I hope none of my pupils will ever halt at this point, for when once the principles of the test are thoroughly understood, it is just as easily and almost as quickly made. The correct handling of astigmatic cases is what builds up the optician's reputation for skillful and scientific work, and forms the most profitable part of his business. As we saw in Lesson No. 13, we can depend, in the majority of cases, that with the spherical correction before the eye, we have the weakest meridian corrected, thus leaving one focus upon the retina while the other is in front. In that case we have only to try concave cylinders placed with their axes at right angles to the most distinct line until all the lines are alike, when after rotating the cylinder to find the best position, and trying a little stronger convex, the test is finished. Although this method seems very simple and easy to understand, yet, to the beginner many difficulties arise which are apt to confuse and discourage him.

In the first place it is often difficult to make the patient comprehend just what you are after, and his answers will therefore be misleading. In fact one of the greatest troubles we have to contend with is the unsatisfactory replies of the patient. In asking about the radiating lines a great many seem to think they are expected to see one line blacker than the rest, so that at every addition of the cylinder they simply name some other line that is black, thus jumping from one line to another leaving the optician in the dark as to the real condition. To avoid this you must be sure that the patient understands your object, which is to get the lines all equally distinct, and then you will have no trouble in that direction. Another difficulty is in determining whether a certain cylinder is not of the proper strength, or if the axis is incorrect. A great deal of time is often lost in deciding this question, which in some cases may shake the customer's confidence in you as a skillful optician. For example he tells you that a certain diagonal line is more distinct than the others, and you take up a -0.50 cyl. placing it before him with the axis (as near as you can tell) at right angles to that line, asking him if they look any nearer alike. He answers that they do not. You would at first thought be led to suppose that you were on the wrong track, and that a convex cylinder was required instead. Before removing the glass however, ask him which line is the blackest now, and the chances are that he will tell you some other line instead of the one he first named. The trouble in that case does not lie in the strength or kind of cylinder, but in its position. Rotate the cylinder in the frame from side to side until the original line, if any, is black again, and always see that your axes are placed in that meridian during the remainder of the test. Always stick to the axis which holds the first line black, and change the strength of the cylinder until they all appear alike. If you are careful in this matter, never allowing the black lines to shift from the original position, you will not be confused, but can make every move count. Copy:

> 155. *In using cylinders during astigmatic tests, be sure to so place them that if there is a remaining difference in the radiating lines, the line which was originally blackest will still be the distinct one. Should another line, to one side of the first, be blackest, the axis of the cylinder is incorrect.*

Sometimes while making a test for astigmatism the patient at first will say that a certain line is black, and in another moment, sometimes before you have time to change the lens, he will say that the line running at right angles to the first is now the black one. When this occurs you may know without doubt that the full spherical correction is not yet placed before him, for the reason of the lines changing in this way is because the patient with his accommodation, is changing first one focus then the other upon the retina. If sufficient convex power is placed before him to bring the focus of the weaker meridian to the retina and at the same time place the accommodation at rest, it will be impossible for him to accomplish this change, for with the uncorrected focus before the retina, he must relax in order to throw it back, and as the accommodation is already at rest it can certainly not relax further. On the other hand if he uses his accommodation both foci will be in front of the retina, and as this would make vision worse he will not attempt it. We therefore have him, as he might say, in a vice, and can go on with the test as easily as if he had no accommodation at all. So when our patients see first one line and then its opposite, black, we should place enough convex power before him to hold one line steady. That is, continue to add plus lenses until one of the lines remain black in spite of him, and then proceed with cylinders. He may say that the convex glass makes vision worse, as it does sometimes, owing to the patient seeing best with the focal interval upon the retina, but do not let that deter you from giving him enough plus to hold his accommodation quiet. The vision will come out all right when the proper cylinder is placed. The following rule may therefore be deducted. Copy:

*156. If in testing for astigmatism the patient tells you that first one line is black
and a moment afterwards says that the line at right angles to the first is now the
black one, you may know that you have not yet reached the full spherical
correction. A stronger convex or weaker concave lens will correct this difficulty.*

I notice a prevailing error with pupils is to depend too much upon the radiating lines in testing for astigmatism. Many astigmatic persons who have reached an advanced age, and some younger persons as well, have become so habituated to their peculiar form of vision that they will notice no difference in the lines even when there is a marked contrast. That is, they have always seen a wheel under these same conditions, and knowing that all the spokes are alike have learned to consider them so. In this case we cannot depend upon their answers regarding the lines, but must try the cylinders with a view to improving the letters. This is really what should always be done instead of trying to get the lines alike at first. Simply use the wheel as a guide to the meridians, and then go back to the letters again, trying with your cylinder to improve them. In this way, occasionally glancing back at the lines in order to keep on the right track, you can make much more rapid headway and can depend more upon the patient's answers. If you have a good test card, one in which there is not too much contrast in size from one line of letters to another, you can easily detect a change of a quarter dioptre cylinder without having to refer to the lines except for occasional hints. The cards ordinarily used show so much contrast in the size of the letters, that a weak cylinder will have no effect upon the vision, but there are a number of cards upon the market, which are constructed with a view to this test, and although the price is usually a little higher than for the regular cards, it is decidedly a good investment for every optician to have one of them. Copy:

157. In testing for astigmatism, too much reliance should not be placed in the radiating lines, but the principal attention given to the best types. The lines should only serve as an auxilliary, giving you a hint as to the position of the principal meridians, and keeping you on the right track by glancing at them occasionally during the test. Of course when the test is finished the lines must be a uniform color, or the correct lenses are not yet reached. In rotating the cylinder to find the best position for the axis, you can also get better results in the majority of cases, by directing the patient to watch the letters rather than the radiating lines.

We sometimes find patients who tell us that the pair of spherical glasses which they have been wearing are perfectly satisfactory except that they can see better by inclining the head in some particular direction than when they look squarely through them. Or they may, during the test, incline their heads to look through the trial lenses, saying that the test types look plainer that way. This is always an indication of astigmatism, for a spherical lens turned obliquely has the effect of a sphero-cylinder. To demonstrate this, take from your trial case a plus 0.50 lens, and holding it two or three inches from your eye, look toward the astigmatic dial. If your eye is free from astigmatism you will see the lines of an equal blackness. Now rotate the lens a little ways on its horizontal axis, that is, tip the upper edge forward, and the lower edge backward, and the vertical line on the chart will be black while the others are dimmed, thus showing that you have added a convex cylinder (with its axis horizontal) to the original sphere. Copy:

158. A spherical lens so rotated that it is looked through obliquely, has the effect of a sphero-cylindrical lens with its axis parallel to the axis upon which the lens is rotated.

Another method of testing and fitting astigmatism is by the "Stenopaic Slit." This consists of an opaque disc with a long narrow slit cut through the center, and is furnished in every good trial case. Having first determined the principal meridians of the eye under test, we place this disc before it, with the slit standing parallel with one of them, and proceed to fit the eye with spherical lenses precisely as we do in simple cases of myopia and hypermetropia. Having found the correcting glass we make a note of it, and after removing it turn the slit to a position at right angles to the first and proceed with sphericals as before. In this way we are enabled to measure each meridian separately, and can easily write a prescription which will correct the defect. It is well to put the combination in the frames, after the test is made and try what alterations may be made in the strength of the lenses or in the axis of the cylinder. Copy:

159. In cases of astigmatism when the patient's answers are confusing, the defect may be determined by the stenopaic disc, which, by excluding every meridian save one, enables us to ascertain the condition of each meridian separately.

In patients over 50 years of age the correction of astigmatism is not, in the majority of cases, satisfactory. That is, in people who have never worn cylindrical lenses. The only explanation for this is that they have been so long accustomed to the old way that vision under the new conditions is very uncomfortable and strange. Of course there are many cases of low degree, and especially those having the axis of the cylinder either vertical or horizontal, who will bear the correction and who even get relief by doing so, but in most cases it will be as well to let the distant vision alone, or correct as far as possible with spherical lenses, and also give spherical lenses for reading, unless your judgment in the case, should indicate otherwise. Copy:

160. It is usually difficult, and sometimes impossible, for patients who have passed
middle life without wearing compound lenses, to become accustomed to a
correction of their astigmatism. In such cases we can only prescribe the spherical
lenses which give the best vision. This rule applies only to oblique astigmatism
and not to vertical or horizontal astigmatism.

Any person who has never worn cylindrical lenses will be apt to find that for the first few days of wearing them objects will appear distorted, or inclined. For instance, a door or window may appear broader at the top than at the bottom, trees may appear to lean, or the floor be inclined. This "Metamorphopsia," as it is called, is very disagreeable to persons of nervous temperament and sometimes causes much dissatisfaction and distrust. It is a good rule never to allow a patient to leave the office with compound lenses, without first warning him that objects will probably appear distorted for a few days, and that it will require some patience to become accustomed to the new condition of things. By describing to them just what to expect, they will not be alarmed at the peculiar appearance of objects, and will have confidence in you that you understand your business perfectly. But on the other hand should you fail to warn them of this before they leave, they will very likely return in a short time with bitter complaints, and destroyed confidence, which all the explanations you can make will fail to restore. I think it is usually better to speak of this just as the patient is leaving, after the glasses are paid for, as many customers are extremely suspicious of opticians and you might lose a sale at the last moment by awakening these suspicions. The distrust of the public is one of the greatest difficulties with which the honest optician has to contend, and we can hardly wonder at it when we think of the innumerable swindles which have for the past few years been practiced upon them by traveling quacks and spectacle venders. We can only endeavor to prove by honest and fair dealing, that our business is a legitimate one, and that we are entitled to the same respect and confidence that is enjoyed by any other profession or line of business.

The metamorphopsia need cause no feeling of doubt on your part that the glasses are not correct, for if you have been careful in making the test, you may rest assured that all trouble will disappear in time. With some patients it only lasts an hour, with others a day or a week, and with some it may even be a month before it disappears. Only patience is required for it is certain to disappear in the end. The metamorphopsia is always more strongly marked in cases of oblique astigmatism than in vertical or horizontal astigmatism. Copy:

161. It is always advisable in giving a patient his first pair of compound lenses, to
warn him of the distorted appearance which the lenses will give to objects for the
first few days, until he has become accustomed to them. This distortion, or
metamorphopsia, is certain to disappear in time, if the lenses are correct.

There are two instruments frequently used in testing astigmatism that are deserving of mention here. One is the "Placido Disc" the other the "Ophthalmometer." These instruments are based upon the principles of corneal reflection, and are used in determining the astigmatism of the cornea. You will find illustrations of both in nearly all of the catalogues. Placido's Disc consists of a large circular disc, about a foot in diameter mounted upon a handle. In the center of this disc is a sight hole, similar to that of the retinoscope, except that a magnifying lens is set into it. Upon the front surface of the disc is painted alternate black and white rings surrounding the common center. By placing a lamp behind the patient, and making an examination of the eye through the sight hole of the disc, a reflected image of the disc will be seen upon the cornea, of an oval form in astigmatism. The Ophthalmometer is based upon the same principle, except that it is adjustable, and more complicated, and will indicate the exact amount of astigmatism present, and the correct axis for the cylinder. The chief objection to both instruments is, that they only give us the condition of the cornea without informing us whether the crystalline lens is astigmatic or not.

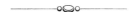

This lesson's examination will be just the reverse of last lesson. The question will indicate the cross, from which two different prescriptions are to be written. To do this you simply take one of the powers of the cross for a spherical lens, and add to it such cylinder as will give the desired result. Then take the other power of the cross for the sphere and write a second prescription in the same manner.

QUESTIONS ON LESSON NO. 16.

Write two separate prescriptions which will form the cross indicated in the following questions.

264. Ver. plus 1. Hor. — 0.75	272. Ver. — 4. Hor. nothing
265. " plus 3.75 " — 4.	273. " plus 1. " plus 3.
266. " plus 3. " plus 7.	274. " plus 3. " — 3.75
267. " — 1.50 " plus 3.	275. " — 6. " — 3.
268. " plus 4. " plus 3.	276. " — 8. " plus 4.
269. " — 1. " — 6.	277. " plus 9. " — 4.
270. " plus 3. " — 3.	278. " — 4. " plus 6.
271. " — 4. " — 1.50	279. " — 9. " nothing

EXPLANATIONS ON LESSON NO. 15 AND NO. 16.

249. If we have in the trial frame a plus 1 D sphere and also a — 1.50 D cyl. ax. 180 we will have a power along the horizontal meridian equal to plus 1 D for the axis of the cylinder has no effect and the sphere works alone. In the vertical meridian, however, we not only have the refractive power of the sphere but also of the cylinder, for the CURVE of the cylinder is at right angles to its axis. Hence in the vertical meridian the power is equal to the sphere and cylinder combined, which is — 0.50. Hence the strength of this compound lens can be represented by a cross the vertical meridian being marked — 0.50 D and the horizontal plus 1.00 D.

250. This, and the remaining question in Lesson No. 15, is worked out by the same principle. Answer: Vertical plus 3.75 D. Horizontal plus 4.75 D.

251. Vertical   — 0.75   Horizontal plus 2.75.

252.   "   — 1.00   "   — 4.00.

252.   "   nothing   "   plus 3.00.

254.	"	— 1.50	"	— 5.25.	
255.	"	— 1.00	"	plus 7.00.	
256.	"	— 3.00	"	— 5.00.	
257.	"	plus 13.00	"	plus 4.00.	
258.	"	nothing	"	— 1.00.	
259.	"	nothing	"	plus 3.00.	
260.	"	nothing	"	— 6.00.	
261.	"	— 7.00	"	— 3.00.	
262.	"	— 4.00	"	— 8.00.	
263.	"	plus 8.00	"	plus 4.00.	

264. We have two ways of making a compound lens of this power. We can use a sphere of the right strength to make the power called for in the vertical meridian and then add to it a cylinder that will give us the desired power in the horizontal meridian. Or, we can use a sphere to give us the horizontal power and add to it a cylinder that will give us the vertical power. In the first case we would first place 1 D sphere in the frame which would give us just the desired power in the vertical. We would then place in front of it (or behind it) a—1.75 D cyl. axis vertical. This minus cylinder having its axis vertical would leave the vertical meridian just as it was but in the horizontal meridian it would not only entirely neutralize the plus 1 D sphere but would leave a preponderance of minus to the amount of 0.75 D which is just what the problem calls for. In the second case we would first place a — 0.75 D sphere in the frame which would give us just the desired power in the horizontal. We would then place in front of it a plus 1.75 D cyl. axis horizontal. This plus cylinder having its axis horizontal would leave the horizontal meridian just as it was but in the vertical meridian it would not only neutralize the — 0.75 D sphere but would leave a preponderance of plus to the amount of 1 D which is what the problem calls for. Our two prescriptions then are plus 1 D sph. ⌒ — 1.75 D cyl. ax. 90 and — 0.75 D sph. ⌒ plus 1.75 D cyl. ax. 180.

265. In the same manner we get plus 3.75 sph. ⌒ — 7.75 cyl. ax. 90 and — 4.00 sph. ⌒ plus 7.75 cyl. ax. 180.

266. Plus 3. ⌒ plus 4. ax. 90 and plus 7. ⌒ — 4. ax. 180.
267. — 1.50 ⌒ 4.50 ax. 90 " plus 3. ⌒ — 4.50 ax. 180.
268. Plus 4. ⌒ — 1. ax. 90 " plus 3. ⌒ plus 1. ax. 180.
269. — 1. ⌒ — 5. ax. 90 " — 6. ⌒ plus 5. ax. 180.
270. Plus 3. ⌒ — 6. ax. 90 " — 3. ⌒ plus 6. ax. 180.
270. — 3. ⌒ — 6. ax. 90 " — 3. ⌒ plus 6. ax. 180.
271. — 4. ⌒ plus 2.50 ax. 90 " — 1.50 ⌒ — 2.50 ax. 180.
272. — 4. ⌒ plus 4. ax. 90 " — 4. cyl. ax. 180.
273. Plus 1. ⌒ plus 2. ax. 90 " plus 3.00 ⌒ — 2. ax. 180.
274. Plus 3. ⌒ — 6.75 ax. 90 " — 3.75 ( ) plus 6.75 ax. 180.
275. — 6. ⌒ plus 3. ax. 90 " — 3. ⌒ — 3. ax. 180.
276. — 8. ⌒ plus 12. ax. 90 " plus 4. ⌒ — 12. ax. 180.
277. — 9. ⌒ — 13. ax. 90 " — 4. ⌒ plus 13. ax. 180.
278. — 4. ⌒ plus 10. ax. 90 " plus 6. ⌒ — 10. ax. 180.
279. — 9. ⌒ 9. ax. 90 " — 9. cyl. ax. 180.

In reply to a number of inquiries from the class as to the best periodical devoted to opticians I would say that The Optical Journal, published by Mr. F. Boger, 36 Maiden Lane, New York City, is the only journal in the United States published in the interest of optics and opticians exclusively. It is a wide-awake, up-to-date monthly and none of the class can afford to be without it. It contains news of the optical societies and optical legislation, as well as a great many technical and practical articles from a large staff of paid contributors. The subscription price, I believe, is one dollar per year, and certainly one number is well worth the entire year's subscription to any optician who means to keep abreast of the times in his profession.

Sincerely,

Dr. H. A. Thomson.

LESSON NO. 17.

Retinoscopy.

IN SPITE OF a perfect knowledge and understanding of the different trial case examinations, it frequently happens that customers come to us whose answers are so misleading that we are utterly in the dark as to the true condition. Among this class of patients are children too young to know their letters, dull and illiterate people, and those having "Amblyopic" eyes. The term "Amblyopia" is given to that condition in which the eye is apparently healthy, the refractive media clear but the visual acuteness very low. "The patient sees nothing, neither does the physician" is the old definition of this word, meaning that while the observer could find no reason for impaired vision, still the patient saw but poorly. It is usually the fault of the retina or optic nerve, either through paralysis, undevelopment or disuse. For instance the squinting eye of a strabismus patient is, from long disuse, very insensible to light. Hypermetropic eyes of high degree are not only under-developed in size and length, but in visual perception as well. In fact very few ametropes of high degree, have normal visual acuteness even when the defect is corrected by properly fitted lenses, and in some cases the correction of the defect does not improve vision even a single line on the test card.

In cases of this class we can certainly arrive at no definite conclusion by any of the subjective tests, and must rely upon an objective examination to set us right. Of the numerous objective tests, there is none which I personally value so highly as Retinoscopy. With this little instrument the test may be quickly and accurately made and the correcting lenses chosen even in the most complicated cases of astigmatism. It is a method easily learned, requires no costly or cumbersome apparatus, and is tireless in searching out every trace of refractive defect. In fact I believe that with a perfect understanding of the principles of this test, and skill in handling the instrument, an optician could, with no other equipment than this retinoscope, a dioptric tape measure, and two or three trial lenses, correctly fit and prescribe glasses for over 90 per cent of his patients. This no doubt appears like a strong statement, and would very likely be criticised by a great many writers, but the remarkable success I have had in fitting correctly by this method, patients who have been proof against all other tests, and had completely baffled a large number of oculists and opticians, is sufficient excuse for the esteem in which I hold it.

A more careful consideration of this method of examination than was devoted to it in Lesson No. 10, would not be out of place here. In that lesson we learned that with a plus 1.00 D lens before the patient's eye to neutralize our distance from him, the light and shadow would move with the mirror in myopia, against the mirror in hypermetropia, and would not move in either direction in emmetropia, but the principles upon which these movements are based, and the different methods of making the tests were not thoroughly covered. There are two kinds of retinoscopes, the concave and the plane.

While each has its advantages, I believe that for general work the concave mirror gives best satisfaction. The movement of one is just the opposite of the other. That is, with the concave mirror the shadow moves contrary in hypermetropia while with the plane mirror the contrary movement takes place in myopia. This is easily explained by a glance at Hartridge Fig. 52. It will be seen there that rays from the flame after coming in contact with the mirror, are thrown to a focus and crossed before reaching the eye, thus causing the actual movement on the retina to be inverted. If however, our mirror is a plane one, this inversion will not take place, and the actual movement will be upright. Now in hypermetropia we always see the movements as they actually exist for rays leaving a hypermetropic eye are diverging and therefore do not cross on their way to the observer. In myopia, on the other hand, the emergent rays are converging, meeting at the punctum remotum, and if the punctum remotum is between the patient and observer the rays will cross, thus giving an apparent movement just opposite to the actual movement of the shadow. If however the punctum remotum is behind the observer, the rays when received by him will not have crossed and he therefore sees the actual movement the same as in the hypermetropic eye. It is apparent then that unless the patient is a myope of at least 1 D the movement of the reflex and shadow will indicate hypermetropia. That is, the movement will be seen as it actually exists. It is for this reason that Hartridge makes the statement that when the movement is contrary to the mirror the case is one of hypermetropia, emmetropia, or low myopia, for so long as the emergent rays do not cross before reaching the observer's eye, the movement will be seen as it actually exists. Where then, is the point of complete illumination, or the point at which no apparent movement takes place? If with the punctum remotum behind the observer, the movement is real, and with the punctum remotum before the observer the movement is apparent, it must be that the only point at which no movement takes place is when the punctum remotum is just at the observer's eye. This is really the case, and with that understanding we may consider what is known as Dr. Jackson's method of Retinoscopy.

For instance let us suppose the patient to be a myope of 1 D. His punctum remotum is at one meter from his eye, and it is at this point (the point of reversal) that no movement is seen. Dr. Jackson's plan is to begin at a distance of two or three meters from the patient, and while constantly rotating the mirror and watching the movements, gradually approach until the point of reversal is reached. This being the punctum remotum of the patient it is easy to determine the exact condition of the eye after having measured the distance at which he stopped. In case the patient is emmetropic or hypermetropic he renders him myopic by placing a strong convex glass before his eye, and after finding the punctum remotum and determining the condition, the power of the convex lens is deducted from the amount.

I believe you will now be able to understand the manner of fitting a patient with no other instruments than a tape-line, a retinoscope, and two or three lenses. While this can be accomplished if necessary, it requires practice and skill to make the test accurately, and I would never advise you to depend entirely upon this test but to always verify the diagnosis with the trial lenses in order that you may make such alterations as are desirable. There are one or two conditions required in making Dr. Jackson's test, that must not be overlooked. We must not, for two reasons, approach much nearer to the patient than one meter. The first reason is that in making the test it is impossible to decide just the exact location of the point of reversal, but will be likely to vary a few centimeters one way or the other. Now as you know, a difference of only a few centimeters quite close to the eye means a refractive difference of several dioptres, while if we are a meter or so away, considerable variation may be made without materially affecting the amount of myopia. The second reason is that with a concave mirror, if we approach too close to the patient, the rays will get to his eye before having crossed at the focus of the mirror, thus giving us an upright instead of an inverted image, and leading us to think that the point of reversal has been reached when it was only the focus of the mirror that made the change. Of course a plane mirror would overcome this objection, but as it is not desirable that we come close to the patient anyway, it will not be necessary to use that kind. In cases of high degrees of myopia, where the punctum remotum is close to the eye, Dr. Jackson's plan is to constantly add concave lenses until the point of reversal is brought out to at least one meter from the patient's eye.

With this consideration of the retinoscope, you will readily understand why it was necessary in the regular test at a meters distance, that we either deduct 1 D from the correcting lens, or else place a plus 1.00 before the eye before commencing the test, and afterward removing it. With no lens whatever before the eye, the shadow would only appear immovable when the patient is a myope of 1 D. At other times there will always be a movement in one direction or the other, according as the patient's punctum remotum is closer or farther than one meter from his eye.

We must always bear in mind that when we have placed the proper lens before his eye to make the shadow stand still, we have not made the patient emmetropic, but have rendered him myopic 1 D. Having accomplished this much it is an easy matter to finish the work, for we certainly know what to do with a myope of 1 D. We simply place a − 1.00 D over the other lenses, or deduct plus 1.00 D from them which is equivalent to the same thing. The plan suggested in Lesson No. 10, that of placing a plus 1.00 D lens over the eye before beginning the test, and afterwards "deducting" it bodily, has the advantage that it does away with mental calculations and possible errors on the part of the beginner. I cannot advise you too strongly in favor of using this instrument whenever opportunity presents, with a view to becoming skillful in handling it, and proficient in searching out refractive errors.

In the estimation of astigmatism the retinoscope is most valuable, for, unlike the ophthalmometer which only determines that part of the astigmatism that is present in the cornea, it penetrates the entire dioptric system and indicates the result as found upon the retina itself. Let us consider the action of the light and shadow as seen in the astigmatic eye.

In the hypermetropic or myopic eye when no astigmatism is present the rays falling upon the retina form diffused circles, but in astigmatism (Hartridge Fig. 72) the diffused rays do not form a circle, except in one case of mixed astigmatism, but form ovals and lines according to the position of the retina. Thus in compound astigmatism we always have an oval varying in size with the degree of the astigmatism, in simple astigmatism a straight line either vertical or horizontal, and in mixed astigmatism either a horizontal oval, a vertical oval, or a circle as the case may be. While I do not expect you to be able to distinguish between the different ovals and circles, while seated a meter from the patient, still it is desirable that we understand these principles.

On the other hand I do expect you to recognize the straight line, or the "Astigmatic Band" as it is called, when it occurs. This is present only when one of the two foci is upon the retina, the other still being uncorrected. In other words we only see the band in cases of simple astigmatism either natural or artificial. At such times the edge of the shadow as it comes into view upon either side of the pupil appears as a perfectly straight line, giving the illuminated reflex between, the appearance of a band of light.

Let us suppose that we have a case of Simple Hypermetropic Astigmatism, the vertical meridian being emmetropic, the horizontal hypermetropic. An examination with the retinoscope will show us a vertical band of light, bounded on either side by a perfectly straight edged shadow. Very likely we will not see both edges of the band at once, but if we rotate the mirror slightly from side to side we will be enabled to see first one and then the other. In this case if we turn the mirror to the left the shadow will appear to come in from the left side of the pupil traveling toward our right, thus showing a movement contrary to the mirror and indicating hypermetropia in the horizontal meridian. If we will now tilt the mirror upward or downward, watching the effect in the vertical meridian, we will see that the band is immovable in that direction, except that it suddenly disappears when all the light from the mirror has passed out of the eye. We have only to place convex cylinders before this eye with their axes vertical (so as not to effect the already emmetropic vertical meridian) until there is also no movement in the horizontal meridian, when the eye is corrected. That is, after we have removed the plus 1.00 D sphere, or, if we had not placed this lens before the eye at the commencement of the test, we must add a − 1.00 D sphere.

In compound and mixed astigmatism we must continue to place spherical lenses before the eye until one meridian is corrected when the astigmatic band will appear as before. To accomplish this we simply rotate the mirror along one of the principal meridians, paying no attention to the opposite meridian, until the desired result is attained. We then use cylinders, placed with their axes parallel to the band, until the remaining meridian is corrected, when we remove the plus 1.00 D sphere and the examination is at an end.

In cases of Oblique Astigmatism the movement of the shadow will not be in the vertical or horizontal meridians, but will take place along the two principal meridians of the eye under examination, wherever they may chance to be located. Even when we rotate the mirror horizontally or vertically, the shadow will be seen to move across the eye in an oblique direction. The reason for this is very prettily shown by Hartridge in Fig. 61 and the explanation given in connection with it. The oval or line, as the case may be, instead of standing upright or horizontal, is in an oblique position upon the retina, so that although the movement is actually following the same meridian as our mirror, the oblique shadow is deceiving and has the appearance of moving along the principal meridians of the eye. In all such cases we should not try to measure the refraction in the vertical or horizontal meridians, but should rotate our mirror obliquely, following up the movement of the shadow, and correct the eye in the same manner as in other cases. The astigmatic band being oblique, we will of course place the axis of the correcting cylinder in an oblique position also. Under the subject of retinoscopy, or "Skiascopy" as some authors name it, we may formulate the following rules. Copy:
RETINOSCOPY.

162. *In Retinoscopy the light and shadow are motionless only at such times as the patient's punctum remotum and the observer's eye are situated at the same point. If the punctum remotum is behind the observer's eye the movement will be seen as it actually takes place upon the retina. If between the patient and observer, the apparent movement will be the reverse of the real movement.*

163. *With a plane mirror the real movement is with the mirror, while with a concave mirror the real movement is against the mirror owing to the rays crossing at the focus of the mirror.*

164. *The observer should never approach nearer to the patient than one meter, because: first, the variation of a few centimeters quite close to the eye makes a difference of several dioptres in estimating the refraction; and second, the movement will be reversed if the focus of the concave mirror is situated behind the patient's eye.*

165. *In using the concave mirror the lamp should be behind the patient's head, for if it should be brought too close to the mirror its conjugate (the focus formed by the mirror) would be sufficiently distant from the mirror to throw it behind the patient's eye, thus causing a reversal of the movement.*

166. *With a plane mirror, as there is no focal point, the lamp is usually placed very close to the observer, for the shorter distance the light has to travel the more intense will be the illumination of the retina. With the concave mirror however, we obtain still greater intensity even with the lamp behind the patient, because all the rays are concentrated again at the focal point which is between the mirror and the patient.*

167. *Retinoscopy may be performed in two ways. First, by slowly approaching the patient until the punctum remotum is found, and second, by sitting one meter from the patient and placing lenses before his eye until the punctum remotum is brought to the observer. The latter method is the one most used.*

168. *If the observer sits one meter from the patient, and brings the punctum remotum to him with lenses, that is, causes the shadow to stand still, he has not made the patient an emmetrope, but has made him a myope of 1 D. To complete his work, he must therefore add a − 1.00 D or deduct a plus 1.00 D lens from those already before the patient's eye.*

169. *To avoid liability of error in the above test it is a good plan to place a plus 1.00 D lens over the the patient's eye to neutralize the distance before commencing the test, and after the shadow has been rendered immovable, take the plus 1.00 D lens away again when the remaining lenses will be the proper correction.*

170. *In simple astigmatism, retinoscopy shows a band of light, bounded by a straight line of shadow on either side, running parallel to the emmetropic meridian. In that case it is only necessary to place cylinders before the eye with their axes in the same meridian as the band, until the opposite meridian is corrected.*

171. *In compound astigmatism spherical lenses are placed before the eye until one meridian is corrected, when the band will appear, and we may proceed with cylinders as in simple astigmatism.*

172. *In oblique astigmatism, the movement of the shadow will be along one of the*

principal meridians no matter in what direction the mirror is rotated. In such cases we must conform the direction of rotation to that of the shadow's movement, that is, pass the light across the eye in the same meridian as indicated by the movement, instead of rotating the mirror vertically or horizontally.

173. After correcting the patient to the best of our ability with the retinoscope, it is always advisable to try the correction with the test types, so that such alterations as are necessary in the strength of the lenses or the position of the cylinders may be made.

———o◯o———

After each eye has been carefully corrected, and the proper lenses for distance placed before the eyes, we next turn our attention to the examination of the recti muscles. The consideration of this subject will be taken up in Lessons No. 19 and 20, so for the present we will pass over that test, to the next step in our examination, Presbyopia. As the practical part of this subject was quite well demonstrated in Lesson No. 14, only a few passing remarks will be necessary.

As the distance correction is before the patient's eyes, he may now be considered as an emmetrope. If he is under 45 years of age the distance glasses will be sufficient for both reading and walking but if over that age an additional convex power will be necessary for reading and all near work, as his accommodative power is no longer sufficient for short distances. We must therefore ask the patient's age at this point and govern ourselves by Rule 149. This done the examination may be considered at an end.

To assist you in your work of prescribing for presbyopia, it is an excellent plan to pin or tack a card in some conspicuous place before you, having written upon it the convex powers required at different ages as given in Rule 149. You can then decide at a glance just what lens is required thus saving time and annoyance. I have also found it very convenient to have a duplicate of my test types written upon a piece of paper, together with the number of each line, and pinned before me on the inner cover of my trial case. In that way I am able to follow the patient's reading without being compelled to turn around and look toward the other end of the room.

You have likely noticed presbyopes reading sometimes with a lamp placed between their eyes and the paper, at the same time holding the paper at a considerable distance, and it has no doubt been a source of wonder to you why they should try to read in such a position. It would certainly seem that vision would be better if the lamp was placed behind the shoulder, instead of before the face, and such would be the case were his glasses adapted to him, but the trouble is that his lenses do not fit him and he is taking this method to improve vision. We know that the pin-hole disc will improve vision in those cases in which the image is not focussed clearly upon the retina, and that it will render vision less clear in case the image is upon the retina. If a bright light is thrown upon the eye the pupil will contract to a considerable extent, thus forming a natural pin-hole, and improving vision in case the glasses worn are not adapted to the wearer. Ametropes who go about with partially closed eyes are endeavoring, upon the same principle, to form a pin-hole of their eye-lids. Copy:

174. If a patient reads best with the lamp between his face and the paper, it is a certain indication that different lenses are needed, for the light shining upon the eyes causes the pupils to contract thus forming a pin-hole in his eye.

In testing patients who have passed middle life, two things are noticeable. First, in hypermetropic cases the hypermetropia is to a great extent, absolute. This is apparent from the fact that when plus lenses are placed before them they say they "see better," instead of "just as good" as in the case of younger hypermetropes. This fact, however, is not sufficient excuse for a violation of Rule 153, for so long as he can see "as well" the lenses should be applied, and the fact that he tells us vision is improving only interests us so far as it indicates that the accommodation was not sufficient to overcome the defect. The second point is in the patient's description of symptoms. Younger patients who are ametropic to any extent, complain of asthenopia and headaches, but in the older cases they tell us that they have been great sufferers in the past but for the past few years the trouble has disappeared. This is easily explained by the fact that the younger patients overcome their defects to a certain extent by an effort of accommodation, while in the case of older patients, the accommodative power being insufficient they give up the effort and must be content with the blurred vision.

In prescribing glasses for presbyopic patients, a great many simply wish reading glasses, being either emmetropic, or else content with such distant vision as they have. In those cases which require both distant and near glasses, we can prescribe two pairs of glasses, bifocal glasses, or give them the necessary reading addition in a grab front frame to be hooked on to the distance glasses. This matter may be left entirely to the patient's choice. You will have a great many customers ask for a single pair of glasses with which to see both near and far, but this cannot be given except in cases under 45 years of age when the distance correction only is necessary. Patients will often insist that their friends have such glasses and wonder that they cannot be equally favored. We can only explain to them that their friends are younger than they, and that it is impossible to fit both distances correctly with a single glass after the age of 45.

In making examinations the record book must never be forgotten. In this book we place the name and age of the patient; the visual acuteness of each eye without glasses; the visual acuteness of each eye when corrected; the amount added for presbyopia; the glasses prescribed; the frames furnished and the price paid, together with the date and prescription number of the patient. The following is the form I usually employ in making records, the letters S. H. A. indicating the price paid me for the glasses according to my private mark. By putting down the amount in this way, it will be impossible for customers to gain any information from the book and any carelessness in letting it fall into their hands will not result in embarassment.

May 1st. 1895.

No. 876. John M. Smith, 55.

R. V. 6/18 plus 0.50 ⊃ plus 0.75 ax. 90 V equals 6/6.

L. V. 6/24 plus 0.75 ⊃ plus 0.50 ax. 105 V equals 6/9.

Near, add plus 2.25.

Rx. O. D. plus 2.75 ⊃ plus 0.75 ax. 90.

Rx. O. S. plus 3.00 ⊃ plus 0.50 ax. 105.

Reading only, in steel R. B.   S. H. A.

This form, although not so elaborate as the system of records in a blank book prepared for the purpose, is nevertheless a quick and convenient method of taking the record. The number 55, after the patients name, represents his age; the first two lines below the name given vision both with and without glasses, and the correcting glass for each eye; the next line show the necessary presbyopic addition; the next two lines shows the actual prescription given, (Rx. standing for "Prescription," O. D. for "Right Eye," and O. S. for "Left Eye"); while the last line gives the detail of the transaction. The name and prescription number should then be transfered to the index, and the entry is finished. The index should never be omitted, for with a large number of records upon the book it is almost impossible to find a certain name in a reasonable length of time without it.

A summary of the routine of examination in the form of a notebook rule will close this lesson. If you will follow out this order in all your tests you may feel that you have omitted nothing of importance and that the examination has been made carefully and thoroughly. Copy:

175. The regular routine of examination is best made in the following order: viz.: Patient's description of symptoms; Observation of face and eyes; Concave mirror at a distance; Direct method; Indirect method; Focal illumination; Regular examination with trial case for distance; Retinoscope, Ophthalmometer, or other tests which you may deem necessary to verify your work in difficult cases; muscle tests; Presbyopia correction; and entering of record upon record book.

QUESTIONS ON LESSON NO. 17.

Draw a cross representing the power of each of the following prescriptions, and from the cross write a second prescription having the same optical effect.

280. plus 1.   ⊃ 1. ax. 90.   284. — 3. cyl. ax. 180.

281. plus 3.75 ⊃ plus 3. ax. 90.   285. plus 4. ⊃ 6. ax. 90.

282. — 0.75 ⊃ plus 3. ax. 180.   286. — 6. ⊃ 4. ax. 90.

283. — 3.   ⊃ plus 9. ax. 180.   287. plus 4. ⊃ — 4. ax. 180.

LESSON NO. 18.

Lenses.

FOR THE PAST three lessons we have been experimenting and drilling in the art of transposing prescriptions, and have become proficient in doing so by a system of reasoning which considers the actual powers of the combination in both vertical and horizontal meridians. I now propose to introduce a short system, by which we may almost instantly turn over the prescriptions in our minds, without being compelled to stop and reason out the powers or draw a cross. Every now and then, some contributor to the Optical Journals publishes a page or two of laborious figures and intricate calculations, which he presents as a short and reliable method of transposing prescriptions, and it is a noticeable fact that the majority of the profession look upon this part of the science as something extremely difficult and complicated. The following method and rule as given below, is the result of my own experimenting in that direction and is, I believe, the most simple plan that has yet been offered. I have never made the method public, nor do I intend to do so, for it is my desire that such advantages as will equip my pupils for better work than their competitors are capable of doing, should be reserved to them, and to them only.

Let us take a given prescription and study the process by which it is changed to its equivalent. We will suppose that we have plus 0.50 ⌒ plus 0.75 ax. 90. The cross which represents the power of this combination is plus 0.50 in the vertical and plus 1.25 in the horizontal. Draw such a cross upon a paper and let us consider it. First what is your authority for making the vertical line plus 0.50? "Because," you say, "that is the power of the sphere and as the axis of the cylinder has no more effect than a plane glass, that power is still undisturbed." Second, where did you get the plus 1.25 that you have placed in the horizontal? "That," you reply, "is the power of both sphere and cylinder combined, because in the meridian at right angles to the axis the cylinder has all the power of a spherical lens, and hence both sphere and cylinder must be considered." These replies are correct, and we may therefore say, that the powers of the cross always represent the sphere alone in the meridian in which the cylinder's axis stands, and the sphere and cylinder combined in the meridian at right angles to the axis. I would suggest that you fix this point firmly in your mind before taking up the next consideration.

With this understanding let us proceed to write a new prescription from the cross. In writing a prescription from a cross, we may take either the vertical or horizontal power for our sphere and add such cylinders as will give the other power. Hence we may begin with either a plus 0.50 or plus 1.25 for the sphere, but as it is our object to write a different prescription from the first, and as the first one used the plus 0.50 for a sphere, we have nothing left but to take the plus 1.25 as the sphere for the second prescription. Acordingly plus 1.25 is our new sphere. But, let us look back a moment.

Where did this plus 1.25 come from? Did we not just determine that that power was the result of the sphere and cylinder combined? That being true, is it not waste time to first place those figures on one arm of the cross, and immediately afterwards transfer them to a position of sphere for the new prescription? Would it not be much more simple to combine the sphere and cylinder, and set down the result as our new sphere without taking the trouble to draw a cross? If you will look over such lists of prescriptions as you have worked upon in the last three examinations, you will find that this rule has always been followed. That is, the sphere is equal to the other prescription's sphere and cylinder combined.

Having found a method by which the new sphere can be determined without the use of the cross, let us next turn our attention to the cylinder. As we know, the object of a cylinder is to correct the astigmatism of the patient, that is, to bring the two foci together. For example we will suppose a case of astigmatism similar to that illustrated in Hartridge Fig. 80, and that the two foci are just 1.00 D apart. Now it makes no difference what spherical lenses are used, these two points will move in harmony, and continue just the same distance apart until a cylindrical lens is placed before the eye. The question is then, what cylinder will we use? There are two ways of getting the two points together, one by using a concave cylinder and throwing the focus of vertical meridian back to the horizontal, the other by using a convex cylinder and bringing the focus of the horizontal up to the vertical. In either case will not the power of the cylinder be the same? In other words is it not the same distance from the vertical focus to the horizontal, as from the horizontal to the vertical? This being true our cylinder will always have a power of 1.00 D regardless of the manner in which the prescription is written, but it will in one case be a convex cylinder and in the other a concave. Hence if one prescription calls for a plus cylinder the other must invariably be a minus cylinder of the same power.

There remains but one more point and the new prescription is written. That is, the position of the axis. In the case we have just been considering let us use a concave cylinder with a view to throwing the focus of the vertical meridian back to the horizontal. To accomplish this we must place the axis horizontal so that the horizontal focus may not be disturbed. If, on the other hand, we wish to throw the focus of the horizontal meridian up to the vertical with a convex cylinder, the axis must then be placed vertical so that the vertical focus may remain undisturbed. It is evident then that the axis of the cylinder is always placed in one prescription exactly at right angles to that of the other. We may, therefore deduct the following practical rule which will apply to all spherocylindric prescriptions. Copy: *LENSES.*

176. To transpose prescriptions, combine the powers of the sphere and cylinder for
the new sphere, and reverse the sign and axis of the cylinder for the cylinder.

I know of nothing more simple than this. For instance in our original prescription: plus 0.50 ⌒ plus 0.75 ax. 90 the equivalent prescription would be plus 1.25 ⌒ minus 0.75 ax. 180, the combination of the sphere and cylinder (plus 0.50 and plus 0.75) gives us the plus 1.25 for the new sphere, while the original cylinder (plus 0.75 ax. 90, after having its sign and axis reserved, gives us − 0.75 ax. 180 for our new cylinder. If you will take a number of these prescriptions and write their equivalents in this way, and then prove your work by the "cross" method, you will find that this rule will never fail you. In case of a concave sphere and a convex cylinder, or vice versa, the same rule holds good, but we must remember that in such cases one power neutralizes the other to a certain extent so that instead of adding the two powers, the result of the combination will be the difference between them. Thus in the prescription − 1.00 ⌒ plus 0.50 ax. 180, its equivalent will be − 0.50 ⌒ − 0.50 ax. 90, the − 1.00 and plus 0.50 combined being equal to − 0.50 which we take for the new sphere.

There is one class of combinations that might perhaps confuse you even yet, and that is the simple cylinders. Suppose, for instance that you have a prescription like this: plus 0.50 ⌒ − 0.50 ax. 180. According to Rule 176 we will combine the sphere and cyl. but it is found that plus 0.50 and − 0.50 combined is equal to a plane glass or nothing, so what can we use as our sphere? Just simply follow the rule and if the combination is nothing then our sphere will also be nothing, and our prescription will read "nothing ⌒ plus 0.50 cyl. ax. 90," or, as the word "nothing" is unnecessary, we will simply write: plus 0.50 cyl. ax. 90. If on the other hand we desire to transpose a prescription like the following: − 1.00 cyl. ax. 180, we will consider our sphere as "nothing" and by combining the − 1.00 with nothing, according to the rule, our new sphere will be − 1.00, and after changing the sign and axis of the old cylinder to get the new, we have as our transposed prescription, − 1.00 ⌒ plus 1.00 ax. 90.

Now comes another point that we have never considered. It very frequently happens that our axis does not stand in the vertical or horizontal position, but is placed obliquely, sometimes at 45 degrees, sometimes at 120 degrees, and so on. The question will naturally arise; How may we quickly determine the axis at right angles to those oblique meridians without being obliged to count them off on the trial frame or with a protractor? We also have a very short and simple method by which this difficulty may be overcome. One's first impulse would be to say that if the opposite meridian of 90 is 180, or double the first axis, then if our given meridian should be 75 its opposite would be 150. But this would not be true. You can readily see that the given meridian at right angles to 5 would not be 10, for 10 is only one mark removed from 5 on the trial frame. We must consider these degrees as occupying certain portions of a complete circle, of which the scale on the trial frame constitutes one-half. As we all know, a circle is made up of 360 degrees, and our trial frame, true to this principle, is divided into 180 degrees, or half the circle. If you will draw a circle on your paper and then draw through its center a vertical and horizontal line, you will find that you have divided your circle into four equal parts, or quadrants, and you will also notice that the straight lines form with each other a perfect right angle on either side.

It is evident then that a right angle is just one-fourth of a circle, and if the circle is divided into 360 degrees, a right angle will constitute 90 degrees. Hence if we wish to find the axis at right angles to any given meridian we will add or subtract 90, as the case may be. That is, if the given meridian is less that 90 we will add, but if greater than 90 we must subtract, as 180 is the highest number on our scale. Thus the opposite of 150 is 60, that of 25 is 115, etc. Copy:

177. To find the meridian at right angles to any given axis, add 90 if the given axis is less than 90 and subtract 90 if it is greater.

By following these two rules the transposition of your prescriptions will be very simple. The ease and rapidity with which you can change these combinations in the trial frame while upon the patient's face, often giving you more space in which to work, and setting lenses free which you wish to make use of, will repay you many times over for the time spent upon this drill. For example, let us suppose that you have a patient 45 years of age whom you have tested for distance and find that he requires − 1.00 cyl. ax. 180. The presbyopic addition at that age is plus 1.00 D. If you wish instead of placing plus 1.00 sphere over the correcting lenses, (thus making plus 1.00 ⌒ − 1.00 180), you may remove the distance glass and insert plus 1.00 cyl. ax. 90 which is equivalent to the same thing.

There is a right and a wrong way of writing prescriptions, especially in sending orders to the factory. In the first place plus 1.00 cyl. ax. 90 will cost you less than plus 1.00 ⌒ − 1.00 ax. 180. Again, even in prescriptions where nothing can be saved the grinding optician has a preference for one form over another, as he is enabled to turn out better shaped lens from certain combinations than their equivalents. It is important therefore that we be particular in making out our orders to the factory even if we are careless in making out our record books, one prescription being as good as another, so far as our records are concerned. The following rule should be observed in making out orders. Copy:

> *178. In making out orders for the factory, always transpose the prescriptions in such a manner that the signs of the sphere and cylinder shall be alike if possible. That is, make them both plus, or both minus. When impossible to do so, then write the prescription so that the sphere will be plus, and the cylinder minus. Of course when the combination can be reduced to a simple cylinder, so much the better.*

> *179. When the signs are unlike, and the cylinder of greater power than the sphere, the case is mixed astigmatism and it will be impossible to give both sphere and cylinder the same sign, but if the cylinder is of less power than the sphere, the prescription may be so transposed as to bring both signs alike—compound astigmatism. If the signs are unlike, and the sphere and cylinder are of the same power, the case is simple astigmatism, and the prescription may be reduced to a simple cylinder.*

In Lesson No. 12 we learned the method of determining the power of spherical lenses by neutralization, but at that time compound lenses had not been considered. The manner of neutralizing compound lenses is very similar to that of measuring sphericals except that it is a trifle more complicated. It is first necessary that we find the axes or principal meridians of the glass. To do this we hold up the lens and look through it toward a vertical line, (a door-crack or window edge will answer) and then slowly revolve the lens, like a wheel, until the vertical line appears unbroken above, below and through the lens. When that point is reached we have found one of the principal meridians, and if we turn the lens around to a position at right angles to this, we will find the line again unbroken and showing the other principal meridian. In all other positions that part of the line which is seen through the lens will not be exactly vertical but will appear to slant in one direction or another. If we look at a vertical line through a spherical lens, the line will always remain vertical no matter how much we revolve the lens.

Having found one of the chief meridians of our compound lens, we move it from side to side in a position exactly parallel to one of the axes and notice whether the movement of an object looked at is with or against us. We then add spherical lenses (plus or minus as required) until the movement in that direction is neutralized, paying no attention to the movement in any direction. We next proceed to move the lens in the direction at right angles to the first (the spherical lens remaining on) and note the movement of the object again. This time we neutralize the movement with cylinders, placing the axes exactly over the first meridian. When the movement stops in this direction we are done. A little practice will enable you to neutralize these lenses and find the axes very readily. You must always remember that a plus lens neutralizes a minus, so that the power of the compound glass is always just the opposite to that of the neutralizing lenses. For example when we find that it requires $-0.50 \subset -0.25$ ax. 180 to neutralize the glass, we know that the glass itself is plus 0.50 $\subset$ plus 0.25 ax. 180, the sign being just the opposite but the axis is of course remaining the same.

To neutralize prisms we do not move the glass from side to side, for the prisms having plane sides will give no movement to the object, but if we revolve the prism like a wheel, the object looked at will also take a circular motion, following the apex of the prism. After determining by this method that the lens is a prism, we look through it at a vertical line, holding the base and apex horizontal. That portion of the line seen through the prism will of course be displaced toward the apex. We then proceed to place prisms over the lens with their bases directly over the apex, until one is found which renders the line continuous, or unbroken. The power of this prism indicates the power of the prism under test.

It is often desirable in purchasing lenses, to be able to judge for ourselves as to the grade and quality. Unscrupulous dealers make a practice of furnishing second and third quality lenses to those who are not competent to judge, at the first quality prices. The first point to consider in a first quality lens is whether it is properly centered. That is, if the optical center is exactly in the center of the lens. Decentered lenses have a prismatic effect which is very injurious especially in the higher numbers. To determine whether a lens is centered we once more resort to the vertical line, moving the lens slowly to the right or left as required, until the line is unbroken. We then notice if the line is cutting the lens exactly through the middle or not. If so, then the lens is centered in that direction. We then turn the lens around to a position at right angles to the first and again cause the line to be unbroken. If the line is still cutting the lens through the middle the lens is perfectly centered. Otherwise it is not. The point at which the two unbroken lines intersect, is always the optical center of the lens.

The next point to consider in selecting lenses is accuracy of focus. This you can determine by neutralizing, noticing whether there is any motion of the object after the lens is neutralized. Of course in the higher numbers, from 4 D up, there will be a movement around the edges, owing to spherical aberration and you must be content with watching the object through the center of the lenses.

Another point is in the material and workmanship of the lens itself. Lenses are manufactured from crown glass, flint glass and rock crystal or pebble. The best lenses are made from crown glass. This glass is clear and white, and possesses the least dispersive power, or chromatic aberration, of any material that is used. Pebble has the sole advantage of being slightly harder than glass, but its great dispersive tendency and increased cost, more than overcome that advantage. Flint glass is very inferior and is used in the manufacture of five and ten cent spectacles. These lenses are easily distinguished by the greenish tint at the edges similar to the color of cheap window panes. The idea that lenses of certain manufacture or material possess certain magnetic or electrical properties, is the outgrowth of fakirs' imaginations. The only possible object of lenses is to so refract light that a perfect focus may be thrown upon the retina with the least muscular exertion on the part of the wearer, and to accomplish this we simply require lenses ground as accurately as possible, of transparent material, and with slight or no aberration. In selecting lenses you should also look particularly for scratches and bubbles. Not large bubbles, but little tiny specks no larger than the point of a pin. To see these bubbles and scratches to the best advantage hold the lens up to the light at an angle of 45 degrees and look through it obliquely. All first quality lenses should be entirely free from such imperfections. A good practical test for pebbles is that they feel slightly colder to the tip of the tongue than glass.

Lenses are finished in different sizes, from 4 Eye, very small, to 00 Eye, very large. The standard size at the present time, is 1 Eye, although there is a marked tendency toward the 0 Eye. I would advise you however, in buying lenses and frames, to get the majority of your stock in 1 Eye. The 2 Eye and 3 Eye are more becoming to children. I think it is decidedly advisable to carry the lenses separate from the frames, instead of already put together, as you can then select a frame which best fits the patient's face, and afterwards set the lenses into it. Frames and lenses already put together have too much the appearance of ready-made goods, and the customer is always better pleased if some pains is taken to give him individual and special care.

It is almost as important that the frames be accurately fitted as the lenses themselves. The pupils should always be directly behind the optical center of the lenses, unless a prismatic effect is desired, in which case they must be decentered according to fixed rules. The study of prisms will be taken up however in the next lesson. The lenses should be sufficiently distant from the eyes to just clear the lashes, and the height of the frame should be such that the customer looks through the central line, neither too high nor too low. In selecting a frame of the proper width it is a good plan to stand directly in front of the patient, and with the frame before his face look into his right eye with your left (your right being closed), and then look into his left eye with your right (your left being closed). In this way you will avoid the errors due to convergence and binocular vision, and will be enabled to determine the width very accurately. If the glasses are to be prescribed for distant wear, then the frame determined in this way is the correct one, but if the glasses are only to be worn for reading or sewing they should be some 4 mm or 5 mm narrower, and 2 mm or 3 mm lower, owing to the eyes turning in and down, in near work. Above all things don't, please don't let a pair of frames go out with the temples cutting into the patient's face. I know of nothing that looks so painfully uncomfortable as this. Just a few seconds work with a good file will open the joints sufficiently to clear the face and give the customer a greatly improved appearance.

For ordering lenses and frames made up especially for the patient, prescription blanks especially designed for the purpose, are furnished by the wholesale houses upon application. By filling out these blanks a frame of exact dimensions may be secured.

In filling them out it is not necessary that a frame be found in your assortment that just fits the patient in every particular and then take the measure of that frame and order a duplicate, nor is it necessary to purchase one of the many forms of "facial-meters" that are upon the market. You have simply to take each item of measurement, one at a time, and fill out the blank in the regular order regardless of the other items. For instance, the first item is the pupillary distance. Out of your assortment of frames find one which is of just the right width. Never mind if it is too high, too low, too far forward or too far back. All we are after is the width. When the right frame is found, measure the width by the scale at the top of the blank or by a measuring card, and set down the distance. Then take the next item and find a frame which gives the correct measurement in that direction, regardless of the others, and so on until the whole is finished. I find that this method pleases the customer more than any other way. To stand up and have his measure taken for a frame exactly as a tailor measures him for a coat, always seems to strike his fancy.

If you have a credit with your wholesale house, the payment for prescription work need only be made once a month. On the first of each month a statement covering all the bills sent you during the past 30 days will be forwarded to you. Although the jobber does not usually mention it unless you do, it is customary to deduct 6 per cent discount from this statement if you remit before the 10th. Send him the amount called for, less the discount, and you may depend nothing will be said. In the majority of cases nothing will be said if you fail to deduct the amount either. The jobbers are very particular however that these prescription accounts be paid by the 10th of the month, and it is very much better to do so. The discount is quite an inducement, and the keeping of your credit with the house, provided you have no commercial rating, is very desirable.

In regulation of prices for the different combinations of lenses and frames, is a subject regarding which no fixed rules can be suggested. So much depends upon the size of the town and its location, the reputation of the optician as a skillful refractionist, and his ability as a salesman, that there are hardly two who make the same charges. I will however give you a list of prices which, though quite moderate, may be said to yield a reasonable profit and will serve as a key toward fixing a schedule of your own. Traveling opticians invariably, and established opticians frequently, charge much higher prices than these.

In steel or nickelled frames: Simple sphericals $2.50, sphero-cylinders $3.50, sphero-cylindric-prisms $5.00; bifocals $1.00 additional in sphericals, and $1.50 additional in compounds; simple cylinders same as sphero-cylinders. In medium weight 10K gold frames add $3.50 and in heavier weights $4.00 to $4.50 to the above prices. If patient furnishes frame deduct $0.50 if sphericals, and $1.00 if compounds, from the above prices—In rimless and concave sphericals add 50 cts to above prices; in compounds same price as others. Broken lenses duplicated: Sphericals per lens 50 cts, compounds per lens $1.00. Skeletons 25 cents each, more.

The examination in this lesson is on the order of a review, as we have now pretty thoroughly covered every point except prisms and muscular insufficiencies. These subjects we will take up in the next lesson.

(End of Lesson No. 18.)

QUESTIONS ON LESSON NO. 18.

288. Case: Mr. H. age 53. Examination with retinoscope shows 2 D of hypermetropia in the vertical meridian and 0.50 D of myopia in the horizontal meridian of the right eye. Left eye with the stenoptic disc shows 1.75 hypermetropia in the meridian at 105 and 0.25D myopia at 15. Write prescription for reading glasses.

289. What is the correcting glass for an eye which can read no nearer than 30 cm and whose amplitude of accommodation is 5.33 D?

290. What will you do for a patient 27 years old who is hypermetropic 2 D but cannot read with anything weaker than plus 4.75? What is his condition?

291. What symptom would lead you to suspect spasm of accommodation?

292. If a child showing symptoms of converging strabismus should be brought to you, state fully just what you would do.

293. Name briefly the working rules in anisometropia.

294. Suppose you had nothing to work with but a retinoscope, a tape line and a pair of plus 4.00 D spectacles. Would there be any way by which you could determine a patient to be 3.50 D hypermetropic? If so explain the test.

295. Could you fit a case of astigmatism with the trial case and test types if you had no chart of radiating lines? If so, how?

296. What will you prescribe for a patient who sees best with − 0.25 when under atropine?

297. In the direct method if the optician is a myope of 2 D and gets best vision through the open sight-hole of the ophthalmoscope, what is the patient's condition?

298. Give an example of a case having Latent, Manifest, Facultative and Absolute hypermetropia, giving full particulars of the manner in which the patient sees during the examination.

299. What is the "Focal Interval"?

300. What is malignant myopia and how would you treat it?

301. In most trial cases the plus 3.75 lens is omitted and the majority of trial frames have but two cells for lenses. Suppose with such an equipment you are fitting a patient and have plus 3.50 sph. ⌒ − 0.50 cyl. ax. 180 already in the frames. You wish to increase the spherical a quarter dioptre. How will you do so and leave only two lenses before your eyes?

302. If your patient is 55 years old and requires for distance − 2.25 cyl. ax. 5, give the cheapest way in which to order his reading glasses.

303. Transpose plus 1.75 cyl. ax. 160.

304. Transpose − 2.00 ⌒ plus 0.75 ax. 75.

305. If you have in your trial frame a plus 0.25 cyl. ax. 90 and a − 0.25 cyl. ax. 180 what other combination could you use having the same optical effect?

LESSON NO. 19.

Muscular Insufficiencies.

WE HAVE LEARNED that hypermetropia and astigmatism cause excessive work on the part of the cilliary muscles. That hypermetropia and myopia cause eye strain through their effect upon the harmony of convergence and accommodation. There are other conditions which may exist among the patients which come to us, and which may cause even greater strain and more marked asthenopic symptoms than any we have considered.

As we know, the movements of the eyeballs are carried on by six muscles attached at one end to the ball itself, and at the other to the bony wall of the orbit. Four of these are known as the "Recti Muscles," the other two as the "Oblique Muscles." As the principal action of the Obliques is to hold the eye from rolling over, we will postpone their consideration until the next lesson, and will devote this lesson entirely to the study of the Recti. These are known as The Superior (upper), Inferior (lower), External (outer) and Internal (inner). Both eyes are similarly equipped. The muscles are supposed to be in such a state of balance and equal length, that when the eyes are perfectly at rest they will be directed in a parallel direction toward some object 6 meters or more away. Or, to express it in a better light, when the eyes look toward infinity the Recti Muscles should be absolutely at rest.

In cases in which these muscles are perfectly constructed and attached, such a condition exists and is known as "Orthophoria," a name having something the same bearing upon the muscular condition as "Emmetropia" has upon the refractive condition. Copy: *MUSCULAR INSUFFICIENCIES.*

> 180. *Orthophoria is that condition in which the muscles are in a state of perfect equilibrium.*

It frequently happens however, that one or more of these muscles are imperfectly formed. It may be that the superior rectus is shorter than the inferior. It may be that the external is attached farther forward or farther backward than the internal. One muscle may be a powerful, well developed muscle, while its opponent is weak and undeveloped. Any or all of these conditions may exist with the result that the muscles instead of being in a state of rest when the eyes are looking toward infinity are really making more or less effort to maintain this position. Such conditions are known as "Heterophoria" implying in the study of muscles, much the same as "Ametropia" in the study of refraction. Copy:

> 181. *Heterophoria is that condition in which for any cause, the muscles are not in a state of perfect equilibrium.*

As Metropia is sub-divided into several conditions, as Hypermetropia, Myopia, etc., so also is Heterophoria sub-divided into different conditions depending upon the muscles affected. The following rules will cover these sub-divisions and should be carefully studied and thoroughly learned. Copy:

182. Esophoria is that form of Heterophoria in which the eyes have a tendency to converge.

183. Exophoria is that condition in which the eyes have a tendency to diverge.

184. Hyperphoria is that condition in which one eye has a tendency to stand higher than the other. This term is always preceded by the word "right" or "left" according to which eye has the higher tendency, as: "Right Hyperphoria."

185. Catophoria is that condition in which one eye has a tendency to stand lower than the other.

This term is but very little used as "Hyperphoria" is preferred by most authors. Right Hyperphoria would have precisely the same meaning as Left Catophoria, because if the right eye naturally tends higher than the left, the left eye must naturally tend lower than the right. We will therefore confine ourselves to the word Hyperphoria, leaving the term Catophoria to those who prefer to use it.

186. Cyclophoria is that condition in which the oblique muscles are not in perfect balance.

187. Hypersophoria is a compound term denoting that the patient is both hyperphoric and esophoric. This term is preceded by the word "right" or "left," thus designating in which eye the hyperphoria exists.

188. Hyperexophoria is a compound term denoting that the patient is both hyperphoric and exophoric. This term is also preceded by the word "right" or "left," to locate the hyperphoria.

Let us once for all get a clear understanding of the distinction between Hyperphoria and Strabismus. One would at first thought consider these two conditions as identical. We would naturally say that Esophoria and Converging Strabismus are the same. But it is not so. There is no more similarity between them than between black and white. They are no more alike than winter and summer. There was a single word used in the above definitions upon which hinges the difference. That word was "Tendency." If a man has a natural tendency to steal, he is not a thief so long as his will-power suppresses that tendency. If he is born with a tendency toward strong drink, he is nevertheless no drunkard unless he yields to the inclination. It is the same in heterophoria. The eyes may have an inborn tendency to converge, but so long as he overcomes this desire by an extra effort of the will-power, he has not Strabismus, but simple Esophoria. The moment that he yields to this tendency and allows his eyes to converge, just that moment he has thrown off the Esophoria and taken on Strabismus. In other words Heterophoria is a tendency, desire, or inclination toward strabismus, which is overcome by the will-power of the individual, while Strabismus is an actual deviation of the eyes, the will-power having given way to the natural tendency.

Strabismus then is a condition which is perfectly apparent to the observer by the deviation of the eyes. Heterophoria cannot be distinguished by observation because it is not a deviation in the least, simply a desire to deviate, which is not gratified. In Strabismus there is no strain because the eyes are allowed to follow their inclination. In heterophoria there is eye-strain and asthenopia, varying according as the desire to deviate is great or little.

How are we to determine the existence of Heterophoria? There is nothing in these cases different from Orthophoria, except that one or more of the muscles are making a greater effort than they should. But we cannot see these muscles in their action to judge of the work they are doing, hence every appearance is the same as in Orthophoria, and binocular vision is enjoyed to the same extent. So long as the patient has control of his will-power there will be nothing by which we may diagnose the condition. But if the will-power should be removed, then the eyes would without doubt swing into a position of rest, actually deviating in the direction in which their natural tendency carries them. There is no doubt that when the esophoric patient, who has held his eyes in a parallel position all day long, lies down to sleep at night, his eyes actually converge and remain in that restful position until he awakes. But when his eyes are opened in the morning, the will-power instantly asserts itself, calling for binocular vision, and the eyes are once more in a parallel position. We must therefore devise some way in which the will-power may be removed and this can only be accomplished by destroying all desire for binocular vision. In this case the eyes will swing into the position of rest, and we can measure the deviation at our leisure.

There are many different ways in which this may be accomplished. If we were to cover one eye, the stimulus for binocular vision would be removed and the covered eye would take such deviation as its tendency indicated. The habit of covering the deviating eye is very common with children forming the strabismus habit, for in this way the eye is allowed to turn without creating diplopia. Covering one eye of the patient however, would not enable us to measure the deviation, hence would not answer our purpose. A very simple method is to place a prism before one eye, strong enough to create diplopia. When the eyes find that they cannot overcome this diplopia, they give up the effort and take the position of rest. Let us suppose that we have a patient in the chair and wish to determine if there exists any Heterophoria. We will place a lighted candle, or gas-jet, twenty feet away, and direct his attention to the flame. We now take a prism of about five or six degrees from the trial case and place it, we will say, over the right eye, base up. As the average sursumducting power is only about 3 degrees (See Lesson No. 8) this prism will cause diplopia and the patient will see two flames, one above and the other below. If there is no esophoria or exophoria present these two flames will occupy the same vertical plane. That is, one will be directly above the other. But in case either of these two conditions exist, one of the flames will be seen to the left and the other to the right of the perpendicular. Having determined the condition of the lateral muscles in this manner we next investigate the superior and inferior recti. To do this we must create a horizontal diplopia which may be accomplished by placing a prism of some 10 or 12 degrees over the eye, base in. The prism base up is of course removed. As the average abducting power is only 8 degrees the patient will now see two flames, one at the right and the other at the left. If there is no hyperphoria present, the two flames will occupy the same level, but if hyperphoria exists one of the lights will rise, and the other sink below the level.

If by these tests Heterophoria is shown, it is necessary to determine the location and amount. For instance suppose the prism is placed over the right eye, base up, and the patient tells us that the higher flame stands to the right and the lower to the left. Is this an indication of Esophoria or Exophoria? This is a question which cannot be answered in a haphazard way, but requires thought. In the first place we must determine to which eye each flame belongs. We know that there is really but one flame, so the double vision must be owing to the rays from the flame striking upon different portions of the retinae of the two eyes. As no glass is over the left eye the rays must enter it without deviation and strike the macula. The right having before it a prism base up, the entering rays will be refracted toward the base and will come to the retina, apparently from below, and strike above the macula. This will give the flame an appearance of being lower than it really is, (the image upon the retina, you will remember, always being inverted). The left eye then, sees the flame in its natural position while the right sees it lower, hence the upper flame belongs to the left eye, the lower flame to the right. If you will try the experiment upon your own eyes, you will find this to be correct. If you close the right eye the lower flame will disappear. With the left eye closed the upper flame vanishes. I wish you would get this point firmly fixed in your mind before proceeding farther with the lesson.

We will now consider the lateral position of these flames. We know that the eyes are now standing at rest, hence the apparent position of the flames is owing entirely to the portions of the retinae receiving the rays. The patient has told us that the upper flame appears to the right and the lower to the left. We know that the upper flame is seen by the left eye. What is the position of that eye that it should imagine the flame to be at the right of where it really is? It must be because the eye is looking to the left of where it should. This is a very natural consequence. If you were looking at some object just at the left of where your friend was sitting, your friend would of course be just at the right of the object looked at. In other words if A stands at the left of B, B must be standing at the right of A. Therefore if the eye sees the flame to the right it must be because the eye itself is turned to the left. To prove this again from another standpoint, we know that the mind always projects the object to just the opposite side from that part of the retina which receives the rays. So if the patient says he sees the light to the right it is because the rays strike the retina at the left of the macula, and this can only be possible when the eye is turned toward the left. By the same reasoning it can be shown that the right eye, which is seeing the lower image at the left, is turned toward the right. The case then is one of Exophoria as the eyes have a tendency to diverge. It will require considerable study and drill to fix this point in the mind, for the fact that the image is inverted upon the retina makes it somewhat misleading. I have devoted a good share of Examination No. 19 to these problems in order that they may become clear to you. A careful study of the one just considered will aid you considerably.

The degree of the heterophoria is determined by the strength of prism placed with its base in, out, up or down, as the case may be, which brings the lights into line with one another.

In the lateral direction we have two kinds of diplopia, Homonymous and Crossed. Copy:

   189. Homonymous Diplopia is that form of double vision in which the image seen
      by the right eye is situated at the right, and that seen by the left eye is situated at
      the left.

   190. Crossed Diplopia is that form in which the image seen by the right eye is
      situated at the left, and that seen by the left eye is situated at the right.

If you will place a 10 degree prism over one of your eyes, base in, and look toward a flame, or door knob, you will have created homonymous diplopia. The prism being placed base in, the rays are bent in, thus striking the retina on the inner side and making the image appear displaced in the opposite direction. The right eye then sees the right image, and the left eye the left image. You can prove this by first closing one eye and then the other, placing a strong prism base out, would reverse the images and produce crossed diplopia.

Another method of determining the existence of heterophoria, is by the use of the Maddox Rod. This I consider the most trustworthy test that we have. It consists of a small glass rod, set into a disk. It comes with every good trial case. The rod is simply a very strong convex cylinder and has the effect of magnifying very highly in the direction at right angles to the axis, and of course making no change in the direction of its axis. If we place the rod horizontally before the eye, and look toward a gas flame twenty feet away, the flame will appear of its actual width, but will be increased in height several feet. It will so entirely lose its original form that instead of appearing as a flame it will look like a long band or streak of light running up and down.

With this disc before the right eye, and the left eye uncovered, the patient sees the streak with one eye and the flame with the other. Certainly there is no inducement to fuse these dissimalar images into one, hence there is no desire for binocular vision and the eyes take the position of rest. If the patient tells us that the vertical streak runs directly through the flame, we know that there is no apparent Esophoria or Exophoria, but if it stands to one side of the flame then one of these conditions is present, and the power of the prism, base in or out, that brings the streak into the flame is the measure of the defect. We next turn the rod around until the streak is seen in a horizontal position. If it runs through the flame there is no hyperphoria apparent, but if above or below the flame, then it is a case of hyperphoria (left or right), and the power of the prism base up or down which causes the streak to run through the flame, indicates the amount of the defect.

Another test for heterophoria is the Maddox Double-Prism. This consists of two prisms of 5° or 6° power placed in a disc with their bases together (see Fig. 1 Lesson No. 5). If this disc is held before the eye in such a position that the dividing line is directly in front of the pupil, the rays passing through the upper portion will be bent down and strike the retina below the macula, while those passing through the lower portion will be bent upward and strike above the macula. As two impressions will be made upon the retina there will be two images seen, one above and one below the actual position of the object. The other eye being uncovered will see the object in its true position, and if the eyes are orthophoric there will be seen three flames in a vertical line, the central flame being equally distant from the upper and lower. If there is heterophoria present the central flame will be out of this position, either higher, lower, or to one side. The advantage claimed for this test is that both the lateral and vertical defects may be discovered at once, although there is no particular advantage to be gained by that fact. For instance if the double-prism is over the right eye and the central flame (the one seen by the left eye) is nearer to the upper than to the lower, and at the same time stands to the left of the perpendicular the case is one of Right Hyperesophoria. In making the tests with either the Maddox Rod or double-prism, it is a good plan to place a red glass over the left eye while the rod or double-prism is over the right. In this way still greater contrast is produced between the images, and the desire for binocular vision is lessened. The flame seen by the left eye will be red while the streak, or other flames, will remain white. It is never necessary to change the disc from one eye to the other, with the idea of testing the other eye. Both eyes are included in the first test, and to change would simply be to repeat the examination. By placing a test over one eye and leaving the other uncovered, we simply break up the desire for binocular vision and the relative position of the TWO eyes is taken at the first test.

As heterophoria, like hypermetropia, is sometimes latent, there is another test sometimes used as a preliminary and is often helpful in forming an idea of the real condition. This is known as the strength test and applies only to the internal and external muscles. For example, a patient is to all appearance orthophoric, and yet has some of the symptoms of heterophoria. We know that the normal abducting power is 8°. If we find by placing prisms over the eye base in, that it requires 12° to create diplopia, we know that the external muscles are 4° stronger than normal and may therefore suspect 4° of exophoria. If diplopia is produced with a 5° prism we may suspect 3° of esophoria.

Having determined by these methods that heterophoria exists, what shall be done for its relief? There are three methods of treatment. (1) Prisms in position of rest. (2) Exercise of the weak muscles. (3) Operations. The first method is the one most generally adopted in ordinary cases, although lately the exercise treatment seems to be growing in favor. Operations are resorted to in those cases which refuse to yield to the other methods.

Prisms in a position of rest, means placing prisms before the patient in such a manner that the eyes may turn in the direction in which they naturally tend, and at the same time maintain binocular vision. For example, if the case is one of esophoria we will place the prisms base out, for according to Rule 82 this will allow the eyes to turn in and at the same time receive the rays upon the macula of each. This being a position of rest for the esophoric eyes, the strain will be removed and the asthenopic symptoms disappear. If it is a case of exophoria the prism is of course placed base in. thus allowing the eyes to turn outward toward the stronger muscles. Copy:

191. Prisms in a position of rest are always placed with the base over the weak
  muscle.

It makes no difference over which eye we place the prism, or we may divide the power into two prisms, one over each eye. For example if we have a case of esophoria which requires a correction of four degrees, we may either place a 4° prism, base out, over the right eye or the left as we prefer, or we may place 2° over each. Or we may even place 3° over one eye and 1° over the other with the same effect. The eyes simply want to turn closer together and it makes no difference which one does the turning. The prism must of course be placed base out in either case. In prescribing prisms in hyperphoria however, the position is different according to which eye is to wear the prism. If the case is 3° right hyperphoria, we can correct it by placing a prism of 3°, base down, over the right eye, but if we wish the left eye to carry the prism it must be placed base up, because if the right eye tends the highest, the left eye must tend the lowest. If we wish to divide the prisms we could give the right eye 2° base down and the left 1° base up, or the right 1° base down and the left 2° base up. The question is often asked: which is the weak muscle in this case, the inferior of the right, or the superior of the left? To this I can only answer that we do not know. There is no way of determining which muscle is at fault, nor does it make any particular difference. If the patient had but one eye there would be no heterophoria. It is the effort of maintaining binocular vision that causes the strain. If we can relieve that strain by either allowing the right eye to turn up or the left to turn down, we have given the patient relief and can certainly do no better. Copy:

192. Prisms base out correct Esophoria.

193. Prisms base in correct Exophoria.

194. A prism base up on the right eye or base down on the left, corrects Left Hyperphoria.

195. A prism base down on the right eye or base up on the left, corrects Right Hyperphoria.

196. A prism base out on the right eye and another base up on the left, or a prism base down on the right eye and another base out on the left, corrects Right Hypereosophoria.

197. A prism base in on the right eye and another base up on the left, or a prism base down on the right and another base in on the left, corrects Hyperexophoria.

198. The reverse of the vertical prisms in Rule 196 will correct Left Hyperesophoria, and the reverse of the vertical prisms in Rule 197 will correct Left Hyperexophoria.

We must however, never give a full correction of the defect when prescribing prisms. The weak muscles are to be treated precisely the same as we treat the cilliary muscles in paresis of accommodation and high myopia. That is, give enough aid to remove the actual strain but leave sufficient work for the muscle to get stronger by exercise, and as it gradually becomes stronger the prism must be reduced until it may finally be removed altogether. Copy:

199. In prescribing prisms never give over one-half to two-thirds the full correction.

200. Patients to whom prisms are given should be requested to return in about two weeks for a re-examination of the eyes.

Although it is not absolutely required, I cannot too strongly recommend you to procure a copy of Savage's "New Truths in Ophthalmology." It will throw a great deal of light upon the study of the muscles and should be carefully read by every optician who desires to attain a thorough understanding of this part of the work.

QUESTIONS ON LESSON NO. 19.

306. Name and define the different muscular conditions.

307. What is the difference between Heterophoria and Strabismus?

308. Describe the different tests for Heterophoria.

309. If with the Maddox rod over the left eye the vertical line is seen at the right of the flame, what is the condition?

310. If with a prism base down on the right eye the lower flame is seen at the left, what is the condition?

311. If the prism is base out, and the right flame the highest?

312. If the prism is base up on the left eye and the upper flame is at the left?
313. What kind of diplopia is produced by converging strabismus?
314. If with the Maddox rod vertical on the right eye the streak is above the flame, what is the condition?
315. If with the Maddox double-prism over the left eye, the central flame is nearer the upper?
316. If the central flame is at the right of its true position?
317. If with the Maddox double-prism over the right eye the central flame is at the left of the lower flame?
318. If it is at the left of the upper flame?
319. If diplopia can be produced with a 4° prism base in, what will you suspect?
320. If it requires 11° base in to produce diplopia?
321. What would you prescribe for a patient who, with the Maddox rod over the right eye, sees the horizontal streak above the flame requiring a 5° prism to bring it down, and the vertical streak at the left of the flame requiring a 7° prism to bring it into line?
322. What would you prescribe for a patient having 8° of esophoria and 4° of right hyperphoria?
323. If with the Maddox prism over the left eye, only two lights are seen instead of three, and when the left eye is covered the upper light vanishes, what is the condition?

LESSON NO. 20.

In Conclusion.

IT VERY FREQUENTLY happens that a patient who is hyperphoric will take on an apparent esophoria or exophoria, due wholly to the hyperphoria. For instance, suppose that owing to hyperphoria there is an excessive tension brought to bear upon the superior rectus of one eye. This muscle drawing across the top of the eye-ball will have a tendency to raise the eye when looking straight ahead, but if the eye should chance to turn in or out the tension of the superior rectus would not only tend to raise the eye but assist in turning it in or out as well. This swinging movement will of course greatly disturb the equilibrium of the lateral muscles, eventually resulting in an irritable condition and producing an apparent, or false, esophoria or exophoria. In such a case it is only necessary to remove the cause by correcting the hyperphoria, when the lateral muscles will gradually right themselves, and in time become orthophoric. So in many cases of hyperesophoria or hyperexophoria the entire cause lies in the vertical muscles, a correction of which will bring complete relief. In case such treatment is not sufficient it will be time, after giving it a thorough test, to give the lateral muscles attention. Copy:

201. *In cases of hyperphoria with esophoria or exophoria, treatment of the*
hyperphoria alone is usually sufficient.

Let us also consider the effects which may be produced upon the muscular condition by the presence of refractive errors. We learned in Lesson No. 8 that with every impulse of accommodation there is a corresponding desire to act upon the part of convergence, and that beyond certain limits it would be impossible for one of these functions to act without the other. Thus in high degrees of hypermetropia, in which the accommodation is compelled to do very excessive work, the desire to converge asserts itself so strongly that the habit of strabismus is soon formed. If hypermetropia of high degree will cause so great a desire for convergence that the will-power is unable to overcome the tendency, would it not be reasonable to suppose that a lower degree of the same defect would cause a corresponding desire to converge although not sufficient to overcome the will-power? In other words, if hypermetropia of high degree will cause converging strabismus (actual deviation), will not hypermetropia of lower degree cause esophoria (a desire to deviate)? The esophoria caused by hypermetropia however, could hardly be called a real esophoria, because it is not due to any irregular condition of the recti muscles. It is in reality a false esophoria (Pseudo esophoria, as Dr. Savage calls it) and will of course disappear with the correction of the hypermetropia. For, as convex lenses correcting high degree hypermetropia will break up the strabismus habit, so will convex lenses correcting low degree hypermetropia, cure the pseudo esophoria. From this conclusion two practical rules may be deduced. Copy:

202. *All tests for heterophoria, especially of the lateral muscles, should be made*
with the full focal correction before the patient's eyes.

203. In cases of hypermetropia with esophoria, a correction of the hypermetropia
alone is usually sufficient.

You can readily understand that with the focal errors uncorrected a disturbance of accommodation and convergence would take place, thus making the muscle test unreliable. If it should happen that a real esophoria also exists in addition to the false, it will of course not be affected by the convex lens but will continue to exist after the pseudo esophoria has disappeared. In such cases, after we have corrected the full amount of the hypermetropia being sure that no latent hypermetropia remains, the true esophoria may of course be treated, but the first course to pursue is to follow Rule 203 and await results.

On the other hand should we have a case of hypermetropia with exophoria, the exophoria would be real, with perhaps a part of it covered by the action of hypermetropia. Certainly if hypermetropia, by creating a desire to converge, can make esophoria appear greater than it really is, it will make exophoria appear just that much less than it really is. In that case, knowing the esophoria to be real, in addition to correcting the hypermetropia with convex lenses, we should treat the exophoria by means of prisms. Copy:

204. In cases of hypermetropia with exophoria, treatment of the exophoria, in
addition to correcting the hypermetropia, is usually required.

The effects of myopia upon the recti muscles are just the opposite of hypermetropia. As high degrees of myopia cause diverging strabismus, so low degrees will cause "pseuda" exophoria, and this exophoria is of course relieved by concave lenses which not only correct the myopia but place convergence and accommodation in harmony with one another. In cases of myopia with exophoria then, as the exophoria is usually caused by the myopia itself, we have only to correct the myopia and the exophoria will in most cases gradually disappear. Copy:

205. In cases of myopia with exophoria a correction of the myopia is usually
sufficient.

If on the other hand we have a case of myopia with esophoria we know that the esophoria is real, because the effect of myopia would be to decrease rather than increase convergence. The esophoria being real will not of course be relieved by a correction of the myopia, but will require a treatment with prisms. Copy:

206. In cases of myopia with esophoria, treatment of the esophoria in addition to
correcting the myopia is usually required.

I could hope to give a more comprehensive explanation of the relationship between accommodation and convergence than Dr. Savage's chapter on that subject. I would warn you however against following all the rules as set forth at the close of that chapter, for, as stated by the author, they are only such deductions as would be resorted to in case there was no known treatment for the muscular condition. The rules are splendid theory, but, as we have three methods of treating the muscles, are not, of course, practical. The note-book rules as given you, have proved very reliable in my own practice, and if you follow them carefully, I believe you will have little trouble with your heterophoric cases.

In the treatment of muscular defects by prisms in position of rest it is necessary to be somewhat conservative. A few authors (Savage included) even condemn the treatment altogether, while others uphold it strongly. The subject of heterophoria and its treatment is really a very much discussed question just at present, and it will very likely be several years before perfection in this branch of the science is reached. However there are many cases which can be greatly relieved of severe asthenopia by this treatment, and until something far better is presented we must, for our patient's sakes, continue to prescribe prisms at times. I would not however have you prescribe them promiscuously in every case of heterophoria that presents itself, but use tact and judgment in every case. Some good practitioners follow the rule of never prescribing prisms until all refractive defects have been corrected and the glasses given a thorough trial, after which if asthenopia still remains, prisms are resorted to. While this is all right so far as conservatism is concerned, still I think it is going a little too far, for there are many cases which give evidence at the first examination that a treatment by prisms is required. The following notes will very likely be of aid to you in doubtful cases, and, although not iron-clad, are good practical working rules. Copy:

207. *Treatment of esophoria of less than four or five degrees may usually be postponed until it is found that the focal correction does not relieve all asthenopia.*

208. *Treatment of exophoria of less than three degrees may usually be postponed until it is found that the focal correction does not relieve all asthenopia.*

209. *Treatment of hyperphoria of less than two degrees may usually be postponed until it is found that the focal correction does not relieve all asthenopia.*

The treatment of heterophoria by exercise of the weaker muscles has been developed by Dr. Savage and is attracting considerable attention. A complete history of this development and a description of his methods of applying the exercise are given in his book. It consists of looking alternately through prisms and with the naked eye, at a flame placed six meters away. For example, in esophoria a pair of weak prisms are placed in a frame with the base in (just the opposite to a position of rest) and the patient directed to look toward the flame through them. This will cause the eyes to turn slightly outward (toward the apex) thus calling for greater action upon the part of the weak external recti. After looking at the flame in this way for five seconds, the frame is raised and the flame looked at with the naked eyes. This of course throws the eyes into a parallel position again. At the end of five seconds the frame is again dropped into place for five seconds, and again raised, this procedure being kept up for ten minutes when the exercise is over. Two sittings a day are recommended and the treatment continued sometimes for several months. From time to time as the muscles become stronger the power of the prisms are slightly increased, although they are rarely increased to a very high degree. In exophoria and hyperphoria the same treatment is carried out, except that the prisms used are weaker in the former and still weaker in the latter, than in esophoria. The prisms are of course placed in such a position that the apex of each will be over the weak muscles. Acting upon the suggestion of Dr. Savage, some of the wholesale opticians have made up a series of exercise sets, consisting of a frame with a long handle, a set of the proper prisms to be used, and full directions for carrying on the treatment. The object of the handle is to enable the patient to raise and lower the frame without being compelled to raise the hand to the face each time. Large thumb screws are placed at the joints of the frames so that the patient may change the prisms himself without the aid of a screw-driver. I have found the exercise treatment to be very successful in several cases in which the treatment by prisms in position of rest did not prove very effective. On the other hand prisms in position of rest have proved a great benefit in the relief of asthenopia in scores of cases. I therefore still favor this mode of treatment in the majority of cases, although the exercise treatment certainly has its advantages. It is my custom in treating heterophoria to begin with prisms in position of rest, and if these fail to bring about the desired relief, to then resort to the exercise treatment. Copy:

> *210. In those cases of heterophoria in which prisms in position of rest are not effective, exercise of the weak muscles according to Dr. Savage's method, often proves beneficial.*

A mistaken impression regarding strabismus is so frequently formed that it will not be out of place to mention it here, although we covered the subject in Lesson No. 8. Nearly all students have the idea that the treatment of this defect is accomplished by means of prisms, and in fact that almost the entire use of prisms is for the correction of strabismus. While there may possibly be a few cases which could be benefited in this way, I have never yet had occasion in my practice to prescribe prisms in such a case. In patients whose strabismus is due to a weakness of one of the recti muscles the weakness is so marked that an operation is necessary, but in the great majority, dissociation of accommodation and convergence is the only cause, and is to be overcome by the full correction of all focal errors. This of course applies to children who are just forming the habit, as cases of long standing must submit to operations. The child should be invariably tested under atropine and the correction of the total defect given. The 0.25 D is of course allowed for the over effect of the drug. In addition to this, the patient should be instructed to discontinue study and near work for several months, and be out in the open air as much as possible. In stubborn cases a weak solution of atropine instilled in the eyes (one drop in each eye every morning after breakfast) is sometimes necessary for several weeks, or even months, to prevent the old habit from returning.

A short consideration of cyclophoria will end our study of the muscles. This condition as stated in Rule 186 is one in which the oblique muscles are not in a state of perfect balance. That is, the superior obliques may be stronger or weaker than the inferior. In such a case prisms in any position would be useless, as the tendency is not to turn in any other direction, but simply to rotate slightly upon the antero-posterior axis. The weak muscles can only be strengthened by exercise, not with prisms, but with cylinders. In order to thoroughly understand the action of cylinder lenses upon the oblique muscles a careful study of Savage's chapter upon the action of the obliques in oblique astigmatism is almost essential. Briefly explained, the principle is this: If a convex cylinder be placed before the eye with the axis at, say 45°, the image of any horizontal or vertical object looked at will not be perfectly horizontal or vertical, but will be inclined toward the axis of the prisms. This can be readily understood when you remember that light in passing through a lens is always refracted toward its thickest edge. If a horizontal object is looked at, rays from one end of the object will strike the thickest portion and be bent downward, while rays from the other end striking below the thick portion, will be bent upward. The image upon the retina will of course be inclined instead of horizontal. If upon the other eye a cylinder is placed with its axis at 135° instead of 45° the image in that eye will be inclined in the opposite direction, so if it were not for the fact that the oblique muscles rotate the two eyes into position to receive the same impression upon each retina, the object would appear double, the two images apparently crossing each other like a pair of scissors.

It is evident then that a pair of cylinders placed obliquely before emmetropic eyes (natural or artificial) will cause either the superior or inferior oblique muscles to exert themselves according to the direction in which we incline the cylinder. We may therefore strengthen either of these muscles by a system of exercise carried on in much the same manner as in other forms of heterophoria, except that oblique cylinders are used instead of prisms. These are usually plus 1.50 cylinders and are first placed with their axes about 15° removed from vertical. After exercising for five minutes by raising and lowering the frame every five seconds, while the vision is fixed upon a broad flame 6 meters away, the cylinders are turned to a position 30° from the vertical, and the exercise continued for three minutes longer. The cylinders are then turned 15° farther from the vertical, thus bringing one of them to 45°, the other to 135°, and the exercise kept up for another two minutes, making a total of ten minutes. This is repeated twice a day for several weeks and sometimes for months. As in the other forms of heterophoria sets of cylinders with exercise frames are supplied by the jobbers.

To determine the existence of cyclophoria, the Maddox double-prism is used. First covering the left eye with a blank disc the double-prism is placed over the right eye and the patient directed to look at a horizontal line drawn upon a card and held in his hand directly on a level with, and at some distance from his eyes. He will of course see two parallel lines instead of one. As soon as he has these well fixed, the blank disc is removed from the left eye, when a third line more distinct than the others, will appear between them. If this central line is parallel with the other two no cyclophoria exists. If however the central line appears to slant down at the right end and up at the left, we know that the inferior obliques are turning the lower portion of the eyes upward toward the nose, thus showing a weakness upon the part of the superior obliques. If the right end of the central line appears high and the left end low, then of course the opposite condition exists, the inferior obliques being the weak muscles. Copy:

211. *The test for cyclophoria consists of placing a Maddox double prism over the right eye of the patient, and directing his attention to a horizontal line drawn on a card and held on a level with his eyes at some fifteen inches from him. He will of course see three lines instead of one. If the three lines are parallel no cyclophoria exists. If the central line slants down at the patient's right, the superior obliques are shown to be weak. If it slants down at the patient's left the inferior obliques are the weak muscles. If the test is made with the double-prism over the left eye the result will be reversed.*

212. *The treatment of cyclophoria consists of having the patient fix his eyes upon a flame 20 feet away looking alternately through oblique cylinders and without them, making the change every five seconds for ten minutes. Plus 1.50 cylinders are generally used. If the superior obliques are weak the cylinder over the right eye is placed with its axis at 75° and gradually turned during the exercise, to 45°. That over the left is placed at 105° and gradually turned to 135°. In weakness of the inferior obliques, the cylinder of the right eye is turned from 105° to 135° and that of the left from 75° to 45°. The exercise is to be continued twice a day for a number of weeks. Cylinders must be placed upon both eyes at once.*

Diseases.

A brief mention of some of the common diseases with which the optician will come in contact, and especially those either affecting or affected by, the refractive condition, would not be out of place.

Cataract is one of the most frequent. This is a disease in which the crystalline lens gradually loses its transparency. It first becomes swollen, then shows dark lines running across it, and finally becomes entirely opaque, the eye of course becoming blind. The treatment is removal of the lens by operation. It is not judicious however to have this operation performed until the cataract is "ripe," as it is called. That means that it must be perfectly developed, otherwise the lens will not readily detach from its capsule and the operation will be unsuccessful. The diagnosis of cataract is accomplished with the ophthalmoscope. One or two dark lines running across the lens is the usual indication, except in advanced cases when the whole lens assumes a milky appearance. Cataracts are usually of slow growth, thirty years sometimes being spent in developing, at other times six or seven years. Both eyes are usually implicated although one is generally more advanced than the other.

The refractive effect of this disease is "acquired myopia." The lens becoming swollen the refraction is of course increased, and if the eye was previously emmetropic it will become myopic. If it was hypermetropic it will become less so, if myopic more so. The fact that a presbyope constantly requires weaker lenses in reading would lead us to suspect cataract. "Second sight," as it is called, is only a symptom of cataract. The patient finds that he no longer requires reading glasses only because he has become myopic. If he lives long enough he will be totally blind. In fitting patients having cataract it is not necessary or often desirable to inform them of the fact, for in the majority of cases it causes worry and uneasiness which should be avoided in old people. Simply tell them that their eyes are changeable and that the glasses will be much more satisfactory some days then others. If their friends are with them it would be well to tell them quietly just what the condition is.

Another disease which is often seen, and which the majority of people mistake for cataract, is a growth over the sclerotic and sometimes implicating the cornea, called Pterygium (pronounced with the sound of the first letter silent). This growth begins in the corner of the eye and grows slowly toward the corner. So long as it does not reach the cornea no treatment is necessary, but when it does an operation should be advised. The nature of the operation is to transplant the advancing end to a position below the cornea and allow it to continue its growth where it will do no harm. The usual cause of this disease is exposure to dust or rough weather. Sailors, railroad men, farmers, and others whose occupations require exposure are especially liable to it.

Glaucoma is a disease in which an internal pressure of the eye-ball exists, the canal or outlet which carries off the waste fluids of the globe, probably being obstructed or choked. The eye constantly filling with new fluids and having no outlet, must suffer a very considerable internal pressure resulting in destruction to the tissues and eventually blindness. The external symptoms of this disease are pain in the eye-ball, extreme sensitiveness to touch, an unnatural marblelike hardness of the globe when pressed with the fingers, and a dilated and sluggish pupil. The ophthalmoscopic indications are: a distended appearance of the veins, visible pulsations of the arteries, excavation of the optic disc, and more or less opacity of the aqueous humor. The refractive indications are: early or rapidly increasing presbyopia (just the opposite to cataract) caused by pressure interfering with accommodation, a colored ring appearing around a gas flame, and occasional fogginess of vision. Whenever this terrible disease is suspected you should lose not a moment's time but send the patient to a competent oculist as quickly as possible.

Nystagmus is a condition characterized by an oscillation or dancing of either one or both the eye balls, usually in the lateral direction. It is very common in Albinos and is present as a symptom in some diseases. Amblyopia (imperfect retinal perception) is often present in these cases. Nothing can be done for it, save the correction of such focal errors as may exist and treatment of any diseased condition that may be present.

Tobacco and alcohol Amblyopia, or Atrophy, is a paralysis of the optic nerve caused by the use of the above stimulants. The symptoms are a sudden or gradual loss of retinal perception, ending, unless checked, in total blindness. The ophthalmoscope shows a pallor around the disc with the retinal vessels attenuated and hair-like. Vision is usually very low, often less than 6/300, the patient should be advised to stop entirely the use of both tobacco and alcohol and to consult with a competent oculist at his very earliest opportunity. Even then the outlook is not encouraging for a great many of these cases are incurable.

Patients afflicted with "styes" are usually ametropic and a correction of the defect will very likely remove the difficulty.

Cases of malignant myopia should be referred to a competent oculist whenever possible.

A hand-book of the different diseases of the eye should be in every optician's library for constant reference and study. One which gives a brief sketch of the causes, treatment and prognosis, without going too minutely into details is preferable for every day use. "Diseases of the Eye" by Dr. H. R. Swanzy is one of the best books of this kind that I know of. "Quiz Compends" by Gould & Pyle is also good. In addition to diseases in and about the eyes there are many "reflex conditions more or less remote from the eyes, but nevertheless caused by Ametropia or Heterophoria. These conditions appear in various forms, as Neuralgia, Migraine, Epilepsy, Chorea (St. Vitus Dance), Spinal Affections and even Insanity. Stevens' "Functional Nervous Diseases" is a book devoted entirely to these reflex conditions, and its pages are as interesting as any romance. Dr. Stevens was one of the pioneers in the investigations of muscle difficulties and it is to him that we are indebted for the terms Orthophoria, Heterophoria, etc. The Appendix of his book gives a thorough consideration of the different muscular conditions.

The following prescriptions are most commonly used for the purpose of a mydriatic. A copy of them should be given to the physician with whom you have arranged to prescribe for you, so that he may know just what is expected of him. Copy:

213. *The following solution of Atropine is generally used when a thorough mydriasis is desired. Atropine Sulphatis 2 grs.; Acidi borici 10 grs.; Aquae destillatae ½ oz. One drop of this solution is to be dropped in each eye three times a day (after meals) for three days. The examination may then be made.*

214. *A weak solution of atropine for continued use, as an aid to the glasses in overcoming stubborn cases of spasm, is as follows: Atropiae Sulphatis 1/100 gr.; Aquae destillatae 1 oz.*

Our course of lessons is ended. The course of study upon your part is, I hope, just begun. I have endeavored to guide you on the right path of study and research in this interesting science, until you would have a sufficient understanding of the work to enable you to continue upon your own footing. I believe that you will now be able to take up any of the books of ophthalmology and read them intelligently and under-standingly. If this has been accomplished I shall be satisfied. I would not have you feel however that because the course is ended our relations have also come to an end. I want you to consider me as your teacher, and I shall always think of you as my pupil. I want you to feel perfectly free to consult with me upon any perplexing questions that may arise at any time, and I shall always be more than glad to aid you in any way that I can. Hoping that you may attain the highest position in the field which you have chosen, and with many thanks for your kind co-operation in making this course a pleasure and a success, I am,

Your Friend and Teacher,

DR. H. A. THOMSON.

QUESTIONS ON LESSON NO. 20.

What would you prescribe in the following cases?

324. R. E. Hypermetropic 2 D, L. E. Hypermetropic 2.25 D, R. Hyperphorie 3°, Esophoria 5°.

325. R E. Myopic 1.50 D, L. E. Myopic 7 D.

326. R. E. Emmetropic, L. E. Myopic 0.50 D. Left Hyperphoria 4°.

327. R. E. Myopic 7 D, L. E. Myopic 6 D. Exophoria 6°.

328. Emmetrope. Left Hyperphoria 4° Exophoria 9°.

329. Both eyes Hypermetropic 3 D. Exophoria 4°.

330. Hypermetrope 1 D. Esophoria 4°.

331. Myope 4 D. Esophoria 3°.

332. How would you detect and correct a weakness of the superior obliques?

333. What is Second Sight?

EXPLANATIONS ON LESSONS NO. 17 AND NO. 19.

280. The first half of this question is precisely like Examination No. 15. That is, we are to draw a cross which will represent the power of the given compound lens. In the same manner that we solved question No. 249 we find that our cross in this case is Vertical plus 1.00 Horizontal plus 2.00. The second half of the question is like examination No. 16, as we must write a prescription for a compound lens that will be of the power represented by the cross. In the same manner that we solved question No. 264 we find that our prescription in this case is plus 2 ⌒ − 1 ax. 180. In other words we have transposed the given prescription into its equivalent, using the cross as our means of accomplishing that end. The remaining questions in Lesson No. 17 are solved in the same manner.

281. Vertical plus 3.75.   Horizontal plus 6.75.   Plus 6.75 ⌒ − 3.00 ax. 180.

282.   "   plus 2.25.   "   − 0.75.   Plus 2.25 ⌒ − 3.   ax. 90.

283.   "   plus 6.   "   − 3.00.   Plus 6.   ⌒ − 9.   ax. 90.

284.   "   − 3.   "   nothing.   − 3.   ⌒ − 3.   ax. 90.

285.	"	plus 4.	"	— 2.	— 2.	⊃ plus 6.	ax. 180.
286.	"	— 6.	"	— 10.	— 10.	⊃ plus 4.	ax. 180.
287.	"	nothing.	"	— 4.	Plus 4.	cyl. ax. 90.	

306. *Rules 180 to 188* inclusive answer this question fully.

307. Heterophoria is a condition in which the eyes have a tendency, or desire, to deviate but are held correctly in place by an effort of the will-power. Strabismus is a condition in which the desire to deviate is so great that the will-power abandons the effort of holding them correctly and allows them to rurn.

308. The plane prism which destroys the will power by creating diplopia; the Maddox rod which destroys the will-power by distorting the image seen by one eye; and the double-prism which destroys the will-power by creating three images. The principle of ALL these tests is to destroy the will-power and thus allow the eye to turn to its natural resting place.

309. In this and the following questions you must bear in mind that when the flame appears to be in a certain position, it is because the eye has really turned in an opposite direction. That is, if the flame appears too high it is because the eye which sees it is looking too low. The flame itself, of course, has not moved. If you are riding Westward on a railway train, the telegraph poles appear to be going East. The poles are really standing still and your eye is moving toward the west. It is just that way in these tests. If the flame appears off to the left it is because the eye is looking to the right of it. Suppose you are in an elevator and that the elevator is standing still on the level of the third floor of a building. You are looking straight ahead at some object on that floor. Now if the elevator moves downward a few feet, and stops again, the object which you saw before is apparently higher than it was. You have to look up now to see it, and hence you say that the object is high. It is just that way in the test. When the eye is looking straight ahead the flame is straight in front of it, but when it turns downward without the patient's knowledge, as is the case when making the test, the flame no longer appears to be straight ahead, but seems to be above. This is because the eye moved downward. In this question the line is seen by the left eye and has apparently moved to the right. Hence the left eye has really turned to the left and the condition is Exophoria.

310. We always see the image toward the apex of the prism, hence the right eye must see the flame high while the left eye sees it straight ahead. Therefore the lower flame belongs to the left eye and as it appears to be at the left we know that the left eye has turned to the right. Answer: Exophoria.

311. The apex being in the right eye sees the image to the left and the left eye sees it to the right (crossed diplopia). Hence the right flame belongs to the right eye and as it appears highest we know that the left eye has turned down. Answer: Left Catophoria (or Right Hyperphoria).

312. As prism is base up on left, the left eye sees the lower flame and the right eye the upper. As upper flame appears to the left the right eye must have turned to the right. Answer: Exophoria.

313. The image always appears to move opposite to the movement of the eyes. Hence as the eyes turn in the images move outward and we have Homonymous Diplopia (*Rule 189*).

314. As the streak is seen by the right eye and appears high the right eye has turned down. Answer: R. Catophoria (or L. Hyperphoria).

315. The left eye sees two flames and the right sees the single, or central, flame. As it appears high the right has turned down. Answer: L. Hyperphoria.

316. In this case the single flame appears to the right. Hence the right eye has turned to the left and the condition is Esophoria.

317. As the prism is on the right eye the left eye sees the single flame. As it appears down and to the left the left eye has turned up and to the right. Answer: Left Hyperesophoria.

318. As it appears up and to the left, we know that the left eye is turned down and to the right. Answer: Right Hyperesophoria.

319. A prism, base in, calls for action on the part of the external recti. The average strength of these muscles is 8°. Hence if they are unable to overcome the 4° prism, we know them to be weak suspect 4 or 5 degrees of esophoria.

320. In this case they are stronger than the average and we suspect 2 or 3 degrees of exophoria.

321. The right eye sees the streak. As it appears 5° high we know that the right eye is turned down. Hence the condition is left hyperphoria, 5°. We also know that the right eye has turned out for the streak has moved to the left. Hence, there is also an exophoria of 7°. The correction would be 4°, base in, on right eye, and 3° base down, on the left, or 3° base up, on the right eye and 4° base in on left. (See *Rules 193–194–199*).

322. 5°, base out, on right eye, and 2° base up on the left, or 2° base down on right eye, and 5° base out on left. (See *Rules 195–196–199*).

323. The left eye should see two flames and the right a single flame. In Orthophoria the single flame would be midway between the other two. In hyperphoria the single flame would be closer to one than the other, and the greater the hyperphoria the closer it would be. If the hyperphoria were of just the right amount the single flame would merge into one of the others, and only two would be seen. To find which way the flame went we cover the left eye and destroy the two images, thus leaving the single image in view. We find in this case that the upper flame disappears, hence the lower flame is the single one and we know that the right eye turned up. Answer: Right hyperphoria.

For our final examination we have decided to use the questions on Lesson No. 18 and Lesson No. 20. Those in Lesson No. 18 apply to the preceding studies on refraction, while those in Lesson No. 20 are a good test of your knowledge of muscle work, and prisms. You are at liberty to refer to your lessons or your note books as often as you like in making out your answers to these two lists, for all of them are problems that will require a little thought on your part to answer.

Quite a number of the questions in Lesson No. 18 apply to the explanations given in the three preceding lessons, although not all of them. In answering the questions in Lesson No. 20 do not fail to bear in mind all of the rules given in that lesson, for these questions are all of them based upon those rules.

As there will be considerable work necessary in making up the diplomas for so large a class it will save time and extra work upon our part if you will kindly enclose the final payment when you send in your answers to the questions. We will in that way be enabled to place our contract for making up all of the diplomas at one time, and will therefore not only save expense but time in sending them out.

Do not send in any answers except to the two lists mentioned above, namely the questions on Lessons No. 18 and No. 20. Your answers to these questions will give us a very thorough knowledge of your understanding of the different subjects over which we have passed.

In case any of your answers fail to reach the required average I will go over them carefully and send you a personal letter explaining where you have made errors and will submit other examinations in their place, and will give you whatever extra explanations are necessary in order to qualify you for the diplomas.

I wish to thank you all for the interest you have manifested throughout the course and the pains you have taken to make it a success.

Hoping that you may all have the best of success in the optical field and trusting that I may some day have an opportunity of shaking hands with all of you, I remain with kindest regards,

Yours Sincerely,

DR. H. A. THOMSON.

Fifteen hundred copies of this book
were printed by its publisher,
The Professional Press, Inc.,
at A. Colish, Inc., Mount Vernon, New York,
the accompanying editorial commentary
having been written by
Monroe Hirsch, O.D., Ph.D.,
who here signs this copy:

This is copy number

262